21 DAYS Cravin'Fit™

Go Beyond 21 Days & Make Fit Stick!

Velma D. Canaday

www.VelmaCanaday.com/21CravinFit.html

ISBN: 0-692-67128-5
ISBN-13: 978-0-692-67128-3

CONTENTS

Part 2: The 21 Hows

Part 3: The Meals

ACKNOWLEDGMENTS

I would like to thank Team Canaday, my mom Patti Canaday, friends Jillian Bridges, Shivawn Hill, Amelia Ball and Kiamkia Pierce. Only you guys know the journey it took to get to this point. Thanks for answering all my calls, text messages and all I'm going to say is #BlueberriesInColor. I want to thank Dexter D. Cohen of Internal Expedition Images for being such an awesome photographer on the cover photo. I would also like to thank Kimberly Clark and Helene Rice for your motivation and support. Lastly, I want to thank Kevin and Marla Elliott of Pure Plates for allowing me do what I love to do every day; Push, Promote and Sell Healthy Food. This book is also in loving memory of my Grandma Velma B. Canaday.

Book Cover Design
Velma D. Canaday; Graphic and Web Designer
www.VelmaCanaday.com

Cover Photography
Dexter D. Cohen of Internal Expedition Images LLC
www.internalex.com

INTRODUCTION

Everyone always wants to know: How do I get results? I want it simple and I want them quick. The results you want are limited to a specific time frame. You are looking for changes in your body you can see physically as soon as possible, and not a day later. But what happens after you get the results you were after? Do you go right back to not eating as healthy or not being as active as you were to get the results?

I don't want you to give up your healthy habits after you've reached that first result. I believe you fall off the bandwagon because you may not understand nutrition and how foods fuel your body and even have the power to heal disease. Don't worry I won't turn you into a certified nutritionist like myself. I do however want this book to educate, serve as a guide, and make you more aware of food choices and active lifestyle habits to embrace.

Chances are if you are reading this book you are interested in living a healthier lifestyle, but you may not understand all the healthy food lingo currently out there. Low-Fat this, Gluten-Free that, Cage-Free poultry, Grass-Fed beef, you will no longer be in the dark on what that all means. I will explain it so when you are in the grocery store you know exactly what you are purchasing. I will give you just enough information to take you from the average everyday person to being more informed while sticking to making healthier choices. And of course I'll show you how to include your favorite foods for occasional treats.

Cravin'Fit Tip: It's not a treat if you eat it every day.

Everyone wants the simple way to eat healthy, lose weight and exercise. Well there is no "simple way." Nine times out of ten you already know what to do. Drink water, eat lots of fruits and veggies, eat healthy fats and nuts, eat lean meats and protein, don't eat a lot of sugar, sodium, sodas, processed and junk foods. I'm sure you've heard this a time or two, or twenty. Do your eating habits reflect that knowledge; NO. So there has to be something more there than just give it to me plain and simple.

I am not here to promote a restrictive dieting lifestyle. That is not how I live my life or what I recommend for others. Restrictive diets are not what you should use or how I have managed to maintain a Cravin' Fit™ life. It's really about being open to new food and health ideas and being diverse in your health. In this book I will suggest that you cut out certain things and you may indeed feel like it's restrictive. For instance, when I tell you to stop eating fried food if that is all you eat, then it will feel restrictive to you. However, if you eat them on occasion, it will seem like more of a lifestyle change than a restriction.

In the practical application of 21 days Cravin'Fit™ I want to explain the What's and the How's. What is this? What is that? How much of this? How much of that? Then also provide the food to accompany the new health knowledge you've gained.

21 Cravin'Fit™ WHATS

1 WHAT ARE CALORIES? DO YOU MEAN DELICIOUS POINTS?...

Calories are the unit measurement of energy. Some of us eat a lot of energy and some not so much. Not all calories are created equal. Almost everything we eat or drink has calories; and of course there are exceptions to this rule. Food companies are working hard and fast to provide zero calorie foods. I wouldn't be surprised if they found a way to make everything calorie-free by the time you finish reading this book. I guess we'll all be eating air in 2020, as long as it's vegan, non-GMO air that has the USDA symbol.

Calories are an important component of healthy eating, but I don't want to turn you all into calorie counters like me; but more so calorie monitors. The goal is to raise awareness, have you pay more attention to caliber and quantity of calories you consume.

Calories are comprised of carbohydrates, fat or protein, and then there are calories from alcohol. Each one of these components has their own set ratio of grams to calorie. This becomes important when you are reading nutrition labels or monitoring your carbohydrates if you are living with diabetes or for reducing your caloric fat intake. The breakdown goes a little something like this:

- **CARBOHYDRATES:** 1 gram of a carbohydrate equals 4 calories
- **FAT:** 1 gram of fat equals 9 calories
- **PROTEIN:** 1 gram of protein equals 4 calories
- **ALCOHOL:** 1 gram of alcohol equals 7 calories

Not all carbohydrates are bad and not all fats are bad. Complex carbohydrates are good and monounsaturated fats are good for your health. I always cringe when I hear people say they are doing

No Carbs. Carbohydrates are the preferred fuel source for the body. Now why would we deny our bodies of a preferred fuel source? Again, you must take into consideration the proper sources of carbohydrates and even the time in which you eat them. As a general rule eat your carbohydrates earlier in the day. This gives your body a chance to use the fuel throughout the day. Your body doesn't require a lot of carbohydrates at night when you are preparing for a restful night's sleep.

Cravin'Fit Tip: 3500 calories = 1 pound.

If you want to lose 1 pound, you have to either eat 500 less calories for 7 days, or workout and burn 3500 calories or a median average of eating less and working out.

2 WHAT ARE NUTRITION FACTS FOOD LABELS?

Sample Label for Macaroni and Cheese

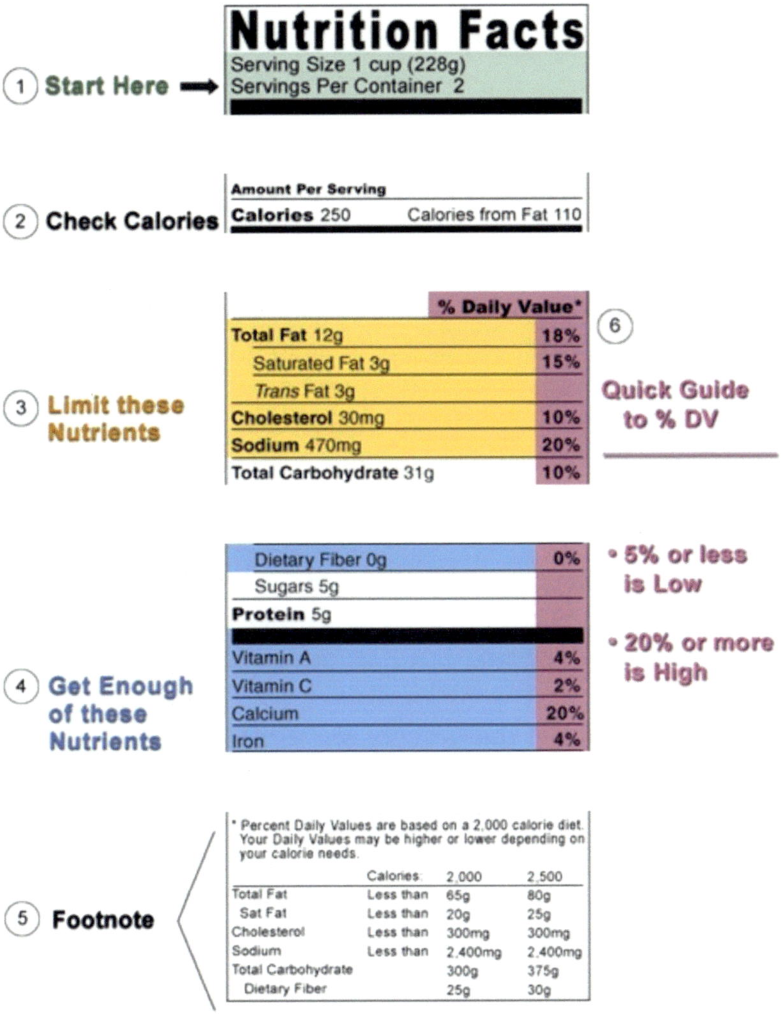

In order to get in shape you need to get your plate in shape. It all starts here and at your grocery store. One of the most important parts of planning healthy meals starts with the food label. Have you ever read a label skimmed over the numbers and said to yourself "Okay that looks good," but you had no real clue what is acceptable or what to look out for?

The first thing to check on the label is the serving size. All of the numbers listed are based on a 2,000 calorie diet. This is not to say all of us need 2,000 calories per day, but this is the base guide. The serving size will help you determine how much of this particular product you can consume. You take that number and factor it into how many calories you are consuming per day if you are managing your weight.

Cravin'Fit Tips:

- **Losing Weight:** If you are trying to lose weight a snack comes in around 200 calories or less
- **Diabetic:** If you are living with diabetes check the carbohydrates per serving. You should also meet with a nutritionist or registered dietician for a customized meal plan specified for your carbohydrate needs.
- **High Blood Pressure:** snacks and sides should have less than 200mg of sodium per serving. Entrees should have 800mg of sodium or less per serving

The recommended daily values provide standardized limits for food consumption, vitamin, minerals and nutrients on a 2,000 calorie diet. You may eat more or less, but that depends on age, sex, height and energy expenditures.

When you are in the grocery store take time or a quick second to compare different brands of one particular item you are planning to purchase. For instance if you are comparing two wheat bread options, go with the one that is 100% whole wheat or grain and has at least 3 grams of fiber per serving. If they both fit this bill and the calories are the same let your wallet do the talking or go for your favorite brand. When it comes to deciding on a lean cut of beef, make your choice based on saturated fat. Choose the cut with 4 grams of saturated fat or less.

- Remember there are 9 calories for each gram of fat. So if there are 4 grams of fat, multiply that by 9 (calories per gram) and you get 36 total calories from fat.

The next area on the nutrition facts label you should pay close attention to is the ingredient list. Please, Please, Please and Pretty Please check the ingredients in the foods you eat! The ingredient list is very telling. Ingredients must be listed in quantity amounts of greatest to the least. You may have to put on your detective hat to uncover some of the names here. For instance there are dozens of ways to hide "sugar" from the untrained consumer eye. I will give you the list of common names for sugar a little later.

Cravin'Fit Tips:

- The shorter the list, the healthier. Unless it's three different types of sugar and then sweet potatoes and carrots are listed at the end. Which really means you are mostly eating sugar with a little bit of sweet potatoes and carrots.
- Healthy Ingredients: Whole Grain, Non-Fat Milk, Organic
- Unhealthy Ingredients: partially hydrogenated oil, high fructose corn syrup (HFCS)

3 WHAT ARE HEALTH CLAIMS?

Health claims are the equivalent of company screaming "Buy Me" "Pick Me" "I can do amazing things for your health." Health claims are what companies and manufacturers put on labels describing how they impact disease risk. For example "Our product dramatically decreases your chances for colon cancer!" Companies will use every claim in the book for their products if you let them.

Health claims are different from nutritional content claims. Did you know there is a difference? It all sounds the same right? This is healthy. That is healthy. When you see products labeled with high, low, reduced, and light these are in reference to their nutritional content so it is a nutritional content claim. This is different than a health claim because it is specifically pointing out ingredients not what its benefits are or aren't.

Nutritional content claims can be a little misleading and used mostly for advertisements to grab out attention as consumers. Companies are to follow the Food and Drug Administration (FDA) requirements for labeling the nutrient claims, but here is what it really means to you and I.

- **Healthy** – low in fat, generally lower in cholesterol and sodium
- **Low Fat** – 3 grams or less of fat per serving
- **Low Calorie** – 40 calories or less per serving
- **Light** – 50% less fat or one third fewer calories than the original version. If we do the math that's 3g Fat × 9 (calories/gram) equals 27 calories from fat.
- **Fewer or Less Calories** – at least 25% fewer calories than original version
- **Free/Fat Free** – food contains less than a half a gram of fat
- **Reduced Fat** – 20% less fat than original version

In the Milk Does a Body Good commercial when they state calcium builds strong bones this is an example of a structure or function claim. Structure and Functional claims detail what a nutrient or ingredient can do for your body.

4 WHAT DOES ORGANIC MEAN?

Organic food may seem like the new kid on the block, but it really isn't. It's just us eating foods they way we used to, the natural way, before modern day agriculture. Now a days we see organic food everywhere, whether it touts the USDA official organic seal or not. The seal indicates different things for different food items. Farmers, companies and manufacturers often times have to spend a lot of money and go through specific farming and livestock raising practices to garner the seal. While conventional farms and companies don't have to pay anything to produce genetically modified, pesticide laden fruits and vegetables. Nor do livestock farms have to pay to provide us with hormone and antibiotic infested meats. Okay back to what the seal means...

USDA Organic produce has been grown without the use of artificial pesticides and chemical fertilizers, irradiation, or sewage sludge. Not everything that claims to be organically grown is truly organic. Look for the seal which indicates that the items have met the USDA'S standards for being certified as organically grown. Having the seal is supposed to inform us that the food source is essentially the same as when it left the ground.

USDA Organic meats must not contain antibiotics, genetically modified probiotics (healthy bacteria), synthetic growth or breeding hormones, most conventional veterinary medications and parasitisides.

For poultry USDA mandates that Living conditions must accommodate the health and natural behavior of animals. Livestock must be given room to exercise, sleep and be outdoors at least part of the time. As you see here, there is no time specification. The livestock can be outside for five to 10minutes and that would constitute part of the time.

The benefit or buying and eating organic foods is having the chance to eat something without worrying what was done, sprayed or modified to it. If this sparked some interest or you want to be more organically inclined, feel free to visit www.organicitsworthit.org for a wealth of information on this topic.

Cravin'Fit Tip

It is a good idea to purchase fruit and vegetable spray that removes pesticides and wax that reside on conventionally grown produce.

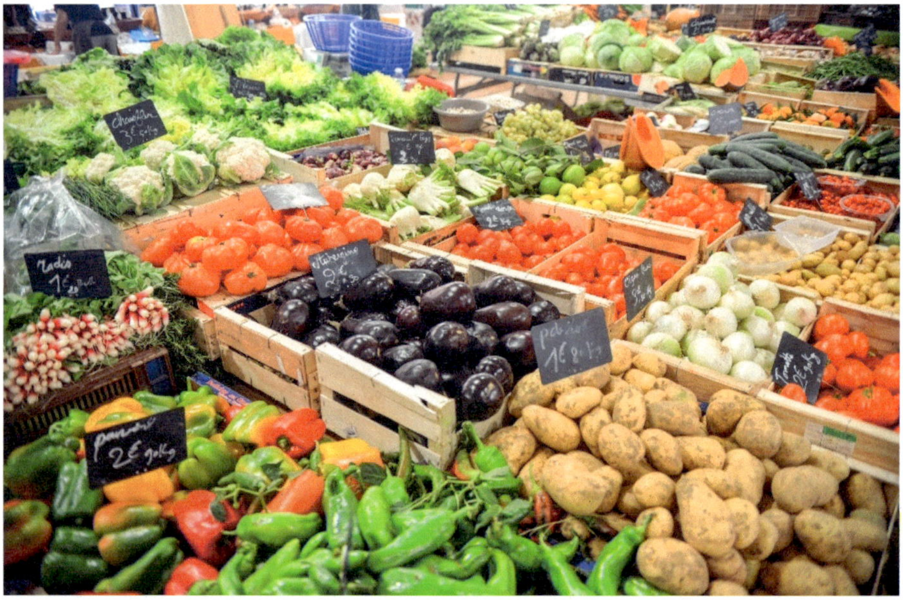

When to buy organic:

- Besides as often as your wallet allows... *caveat:* you don't have to switch to a 100% organic diet right from the start. Eating an apple is always better than eating a whole row of Oreo cookies or a bag of chips; conventionally grown and all.
- Be on the look at for sales at your local grocer. You may be able to snag a bag of Organic Spinach or Kale for $3.50. This price is right on average coming in at the same cost of the conventionally grown counterpart.
- Fruits and veggies that have thin skins and leafy produce

where dirt, dust and parasites can be hiding in the wake

- Please note an Organic Oreo is still an Oreo. Call it Organic Junk if you will...

Quick List of Items to Purchase Organic			
Apples	Imported grapes	Oatmeal	Rice
Apricots	Green beans	Parsley	Salad Greens
Baby food	Eggs	Pecans	Soy Milk
Beef	Juice	Peaches	Spinach
Bell pepper	Kale	Peanuts	Strawberries
Cherries	Swiss chard	Peanut Butter	Tofu
Chicken	Lemons/Limes	Pears	Tomato Sauce
Collard greens	Lettuce	Plums	Turnips
Cucumbers	Milk	Potatoes	Wheat Flour
Figs	Nectarines	Pumpkins	

5 WHAT IS GMO?

GMO is an acronym for Genetically Modified Organism. A genetically modified organism is an organism whose genetic makeup has been altered using genetic engineering techniques. A GMO is a plant or animal that has been genetically changed by scientists to improve its ability to grow in non-native environments, resist pests, endure extreme weather conditions, yield more food (like milk in cows), or display other desired characteristics. In other words a GMO is a new version of a food, plant or animal created through engineering, it's DNA has been changed. Companies are not required by law to label their products genetically modified, so we have no way of knowing. Unless it's specifically labeled no GMO's or non GMO.

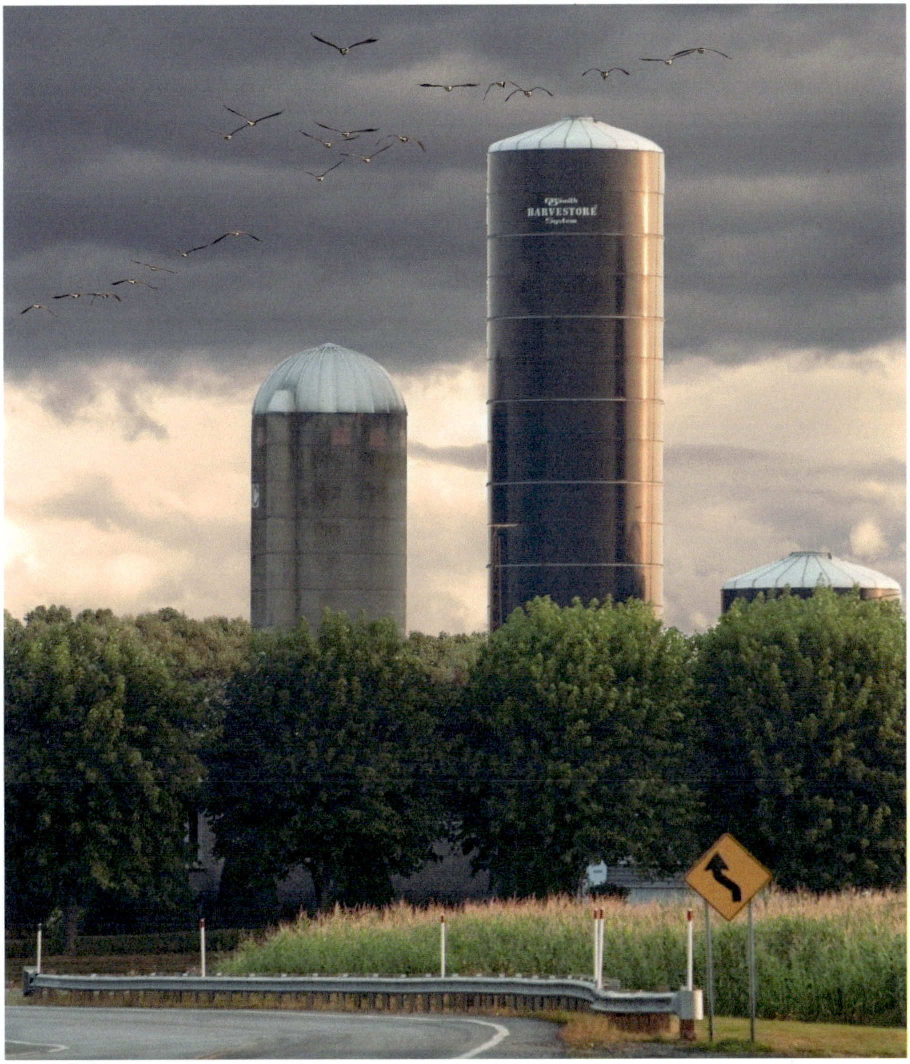
HARVESTORE

6 WHAT IS LOCALLY GROWN FOOD?

If you want to be uber healthy and take it up a notch then you should only eat organic, free-range, grass-fed, certified humanely raised and consume locally grown food. Then if you want to add morals and ethics in the mix go vegan.

The House of the United States legislative branch voted 300 to 131 in June of 2015 to remove the country-of-origin label from meat. You as the consumer will no longer have all the information about the food you are consuming. It is also important to note that not all countries have the same standards when it comes to farming and livestock practices. This can make you do one of three things; become a vegan, a vegetarian or flock to local farms. Doing the latter is great for the economy and better for your health. The meat from a local farm is fresher, has more nutrients and did not travel one million miles to your dinner table.

Food is considered locally grown if it was sourced from within 100 miles of the place you are consuming it. The longer the travel from farm to plate, the more preservatives and irradiation are in the food. Irradiation is where food is exposed to radiation. Radiation reduces and sometimes eliminates microorganisms and insects. This process increases the shelf life and makes the food safer for the consumer.

Top reasons foods are irradiated:

1. Prevent of Foodborne Illness
2. Control Insects
3. Delay of Sprouting and Ripening
4. Sterilization

7 WHAT IS CLEAN EATING?

Is it a diet? Is it just making sure you wash all of you food prior to eating? What is it? Clean eating means eating food as close to its natural state as possible. It also encompasses food preparation methods. This eating lifestyle is similar to what doctors regularly recommended.

- Eat 3 meals and 2-3 snacks daily
- Eat complex carbohydrates -- whole grains
- Avoiding processed and refined foods. You know the whites; flour, sugar, bread and pasta
- No trans fat, no fried foods, not too much sugar
- No preservatives, additives
- Eat healthy fats

8 WHAT IS PALEO?

The Paleolithic diet is based upon what our ancestors hunted, gathered and ate to survive. Have you ever heard of the caveman diet? Well this is it. Resolving to eat only foods a caveman would find in his natural habitat. This consists of fruits, vegetables, nuts, fish, eggs, healthy fats and grass-fed meats. In today's modern diet this would mean eliminating all processed foods, grains, legumes, processed sugars, processed oils and dairy. These are the by-products of agriculture and the industrial revolution.

9 WHAT DOES IT MEAN TO BE VEGAN?

Vegan in a nutshell it is a diet that it is 100% plant-based. No wiggle room here. Individuals who are vegan do not consume any animal products or by-products. Some transition to this diet for more than their health. They transition for the health of animals and planet earth.

The upside of eating proteins strictly from plant sources are that you also get fiber, vitamins, minerals and phytochemicals. You cannot get those from animal protein, albeit animal protein is a complete protein. Another benefit is that going vegan can cut your grocery bill down. You will no longer have to buy costly cuts of top choice meats. Instead you would be buying vegetable proteins, dark leafy greens, rice, potatoes, fruits, nuts and seeds.

Transition Steps to Vegan

1. Eat an all vegetarian diet first
2. Do your homework, research the foods you can eat, recipes and preparation methods. There are a number of vegan options in the meal section of this book.
3. Add more greens
4. Replace animal proteins with plant proteins
5. Replace dairy with plant/nut milks and cheese substitutes
6. Replace overly processed foods with minimally cooked whole plant foods
7. Replace processed sugars with fruits and fruit juices in recipes
8. Replace extracted oils with foods that have oils in them
9. Replace sodium with citrus juices, sodium-free dried vegetables and other seasonings
10. Eat 100% Whole Grains
11. Eat 3-5 servings of fruit per day
12. Eat 1oz of raw nuts and seeds per day

Stick with it Vegan

- Remix your Favs – yes find out how to make vegan mac-n-cheese. It's always a good idea to start with dishes you love then turn them into vegan creations

- Be open to new foods – well you've up and done it now, you cut out all animal foods and by-products now what? You have to find new foods to experience and enjoy. Let the vegan journey begin! Pinterest is a good place to look for quick and easy recipes.
- Begin to love tofu and tempeh these are the main protein swap outs when you think vegan, and for good reason. They are quite adaptable to any recipe, flavor or preparation.
- Make new vegan friends so you can learn, share and be inspired by other individuals who share your new eating lifestyle. Potluck anyone?

10 WHAT IS FREE RANGE?

The free range classification is somewhat ambiguous. The USDA states livestock must have access to the outdoors. It fails at providing specifications about the environment in which this should occur. The livestock could be held in cages, kooked up and inside of buildings that have retractable roofs and this would still fall under free range. Simply because the roof was open that constitutes they have access to the outside. While the livestock may have received access they did not actually go outside to be free on the range. Not so "free range" hunh?

There are companies who actually allow the livestock to roam freely and get fresh air. Most local farms welcome visitors and are happy to answer questions about their methods. To find local farms go to www.localharvest.org and for organic farms go to www.localharvest.org/organic-farms.

11 WHAT IS GRASS-FED?

Grass-fed sounds simple enough right? It means animals were fed more of the traditional foods they were designed to eat; more grass and less grains and corn. This does not mean it is 100% grass-fed nor does it mean it's organic. However, grass-fed meat tends to be lower in fat and higher in omega-3 fatty acids. Grass-feeding livestock is one of the best ways to feed by allowing them to graze in a pasture or field. This is their natural behavior. Allowing them to get exercise and fresh air ensures a lifestyle originally designed for them to live.

Cravin'Fit Tip

When selecting beef or pork look for the words loin or round on the label. These cuts are lean. If you see visible fat, trim it before preparation.

12 WHAT IS CERTIFIED HUMANE?

Certified humane foods mean livestock have lived as closely as possible to the way they would have naturally on any farm pre agriculture days. Animals live in an open space where they wander, graze and are free of claustrophobic environments. Claustrophobic environments include cages and shelters. These animals have not been injected with hormones and antibiotics. Also, livestock are butchered quickly and painlessly to limit stress.

13 WHAT IS FARM-RAISED AND WILD-CAUGHT SEAFOOD?

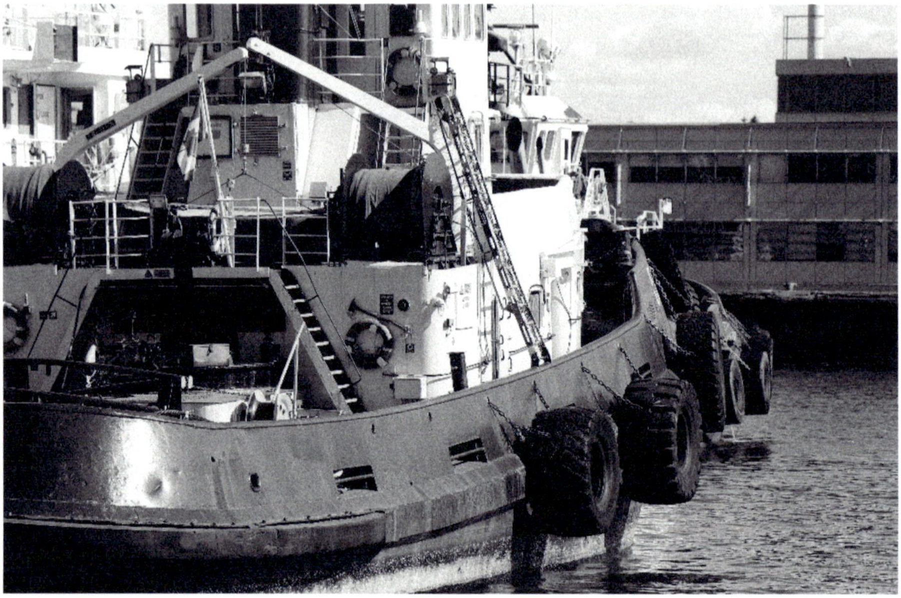

The most common farm raised fish are catfish, tilapia and salmon. Simply put wild-caught seafood is seafood caught in its natural environment by fishermen. Farm-raised seafood is grown in pens immersed in ponds, lakes and salt water. I would like to think farm-raised seafood is the result of over fished waters and the declining number of fish in the sea. Who knows this for sure, or is it more company practices to increase profits and decrease overhead?

Seafood is a-la-king, top of the charts, when it comes to the healthy fats. They are high in protein and omega-3 fatty acids. They are packed with vitamins and minerals that make our hearts healthier and brains stronger. It is recommended to consume fish at least three times a week. That can help out with your meal planning; now you have to figure out the other 4 days.

14 WHAT IS GLUTEN AND GLUTEN-FREE?

Gluten is protein that is present in wheat, barley, oats and rye. It is the glue that holds food together. It helps dough rise and gives baked goods its chewy texture. For some people it can be hard or impossible to digest and can also cause inflammation in the organs of the body. Gluten also encourages the body to hold onto water weight, which explains why people who eat a gluten-free diet report being relieved of bloating.

Eating gluten-free food is easier today than it was in the past. More and more companies are making gluten-free goodies. When you see an item with a gluten-free label it means the protein gluten is not in the product. You can't just stop there, cross contamination matters. It is especially important for individuals who have celiac disease or those who are gluten intolerant to eat a 100% gluten-free diet.

Celiac disease is an autoimmune disorder that occurs in genetically pre-disposed people where ingesting gluten leads to damage in the small intestine. Gluten present in food does not allow the celiac's body to absorb vital nutrients. We eat to live, so imagine eating to satisfy your hunger, the physiological need to eat, and give your body proper nutrition but it doesn't nourish you at all. In this case there would no need to eat if the body couldn't receive the proper nourishment from food. This as you could imagine leads to a multitude of deficiencies in the body. This would greatly affects the immune system, bone health and could cause numerous ailments and diseases including type 1 diabetes, osteoporosis, arthritis and intestinal cancers.

Should you transition to a gluten-free diet? Well that really all depends if you have stomach pains and discomfort that you may not know the cause of. For example you are uncomfortable and experience stomach pains after eating foods containing gluten. I don't follow a 100% gluten free diet. I do however eat a great deal of foods without gluten. Not quite sure I can give bread up, but I do eat sprouted versions such as Ezekiel bread.

Most foods are naturally gluten-free and you don't even know it. That apple a day is an example. Apples are gluten-free and you've been eating them all your life, so thumbs up to you! You were ahead of the game all along. You can find more information and a multitude of resources on the topic by visiting http://celiac.org.

15 WHAT IS DETOX?

Outside of organs that naturally detox such as the liver, colon and kidney, detoxing is ridding the body of poisonous substances. In terms of nutrition that includes processed foods, refined sugars, and chemical additives. Detoxing allows your body and organs to reset and do their jobs more efficiently. As a result of eliminating toxins this also eases the digestion process.

Your natural detoxing liver is designed to filter toxic substances contained in foods from passing into your blood stream. The colon has bacteria that produce both healthy and unhealthy chemicals. The colons job is to flush toxins out before they fester and cause internal damage. It is important to get sufficient amounts of fibrous foods to keep your colon running smoothly. Lastly, kidneys work non-stop by filtering your blood and getting rid of toxins via urine.

The main purpose of a detox is to spend a period of time cleaning up your diet and eating foods that promote the excretion of stored toxins and water. A detox can help you crave more healthy foods and the feeling of being healthy. During your detox you will have a more restrictive diet than normal, but this isn't something you will continue everyday of your life, so it is okay for a short period of time.

16 WHAT IS A CLEANSE?

Cleanse is the way you detox. Often times the terms are used similarly and interchangeably. In terms of food consumption you can either do a juice cleanse or a food cleanse. Cleanses can be beneficial if you do them for a short period of time, say 2-3 days. Touted benefits are improved digestive function, ease of elimination of waste and boosted energy levels. A cleanse is done to relieve the body of heavy digestive periods. Cleansing in a sense gives the system a break from extra food, bad foods and toxin overload.

You can lose weight by doing a cleanse. The lost weight is mostly water weight. Also if you do it for extended periods of time you lose muscle mass. My suggestion is to use this as a jumpstart to healthy living and when you want rid your system of unhealthy food consumption.

Cravin'Fit Tip

Eat grapefruit, lemon and lime citrus juice regularly to help cleanse the body.

17 WHAT IS JUICING?

Green Juice, Beet Juice, Ginger Orange Juice they all have really nice names, but is juice all you get? Juicing is where juice is extracted from fruits or vegetables. This can be done using a juicer or juice press. There are several juicers on the market today. They range from simple and get the job done to the fancy schmancy I-can-make-hummus too types.

Nutrients are more easily absorbed via juicing versus blending. The pulp and fiber have been eliminated in the process leaving only liquid, or juice as we call it. Juice fills up the stomach and delivers a cup load of nutrients almost instantly. While juice fills the stomach you feel less full because the fiber has been removed.

Juicing for a specific number of days has its benefits. Have you heard of anyone juicing for 365 days? I'm sure you haven't Everyday life doesn't make that possible. Let it be the jumpstart you need to pump your insides with the good stuff.

18 WHAT IS BLENDING?

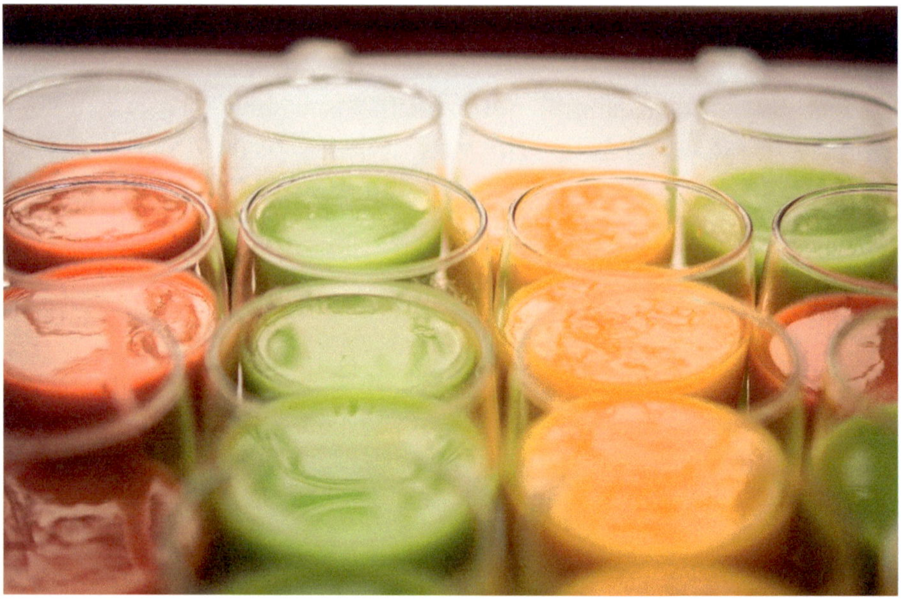

Blenders blend ingredients into a smooth liquid while keeping the fiber intact. It usually produces thicker liquid and has more texture than drinks produced from a juicer. The yield from a blender is not pure juice, but the fiber in it will help you feel fuller. This is also the best way to make awesome smoothies and protein shakes. I included a few good ones in the meal section of the book. I can't wait for you to try 'Don't Take Me for Granate Smoothie.'

19 WHAT IS ALKALINE AND WHAT DOES IT HAVE TO DO WITH FOOD AND BODY?

Alkaline is specific to pH levels. pH is potential hydrogen. Our bodies uses hydrogen to keep cells hydrated, transport nutrients, eliminate toxins and waste, lubricate joints and helps our immune system fight off harmful microbes. In addition to all of those great things, hydrogen also helps the body create more energy and protects it from free radical damage.

The pH scale ranges from 1-14, a quick science lesson here. 7 is neutral on the pH Scale. Acidic is less than 7. Alkaline is greater than 7.

The ideal body alkalinity is 7.3-7.45 on the 14 point scale. To test your pH level you can purchase litmus paper from the pharmacy.

When your body is alkaline it is in the healthiest state it can be. This is where all body functions and metabolism are running at their best. You may have seen alkaline water on the shelves or someone with a bottle and wondered if there is any real difference. The benefit to drinking this water is that it helps balance you from the inside out. It is especially beneficial for individuals who do not consume vegetables or get the daily recommended servings.

Cravin'Fit Tip

Drinking 1 tablespoon diluted in an 8 ounce glass of water can aid in balancing your pH levels. Do this first thing in the morning before you eat anything and definitely after you brush your teeth!

20 WHAT ARE SUPERFOODS?

While there is no scientific definition for this term and more of a term used in marketing and on food labels. Foods labeled as superfoods are more functional than super. Meaning the properties of a particular food go beyond meeting the basic nutritional needs of the body. Their components help promote a particular function within the body. For instance, dark chocolate is considered a "superfood" because of the flavonoids and polyphenols which improves vascular health. Polyphenols are plentiful amounts of micronutrients available in foods which help ward off cancer and cardiovascular diseases. Stick to about 100 calories a day of the dark chocolate superfood. Foods in this newly created buzzword category have extra doses of antioxidants, vitamins, minerals and provide numerous health benefits.

Here's a short list of 20 Superfoods:

- Acai – weight loss and anti-aging
- Apples - fiber
- Avocados – healthy fats
- Beans – high in protein, fiber, folate and magnesium, low in cholesterol
- Blueberries – fiber and vitamin C
- Broccoli – vitamin C and folate
- Cacao (Nibs/Powder/etc) – flavonoids. ***Tip:*** buy the raw or non-alkalized version which hasn't been processed and still has all phytonutrients and antioxidants intact.
- Chia seeds– essential fatty acids
- Dark Chocolate - Polyphenols
- Extra Virgin Olive Oil
- Garlic – helps with high blood pressure
- Goji Berries – vitamin C
- Greek Yogurt – has more protein than regular yogurt and probiotics which is healthy bacteria
- Green Tea – antioxidants and EGCG (Epigallocatechin gallate) a phytochemical that slows irregular cell growth

- Hemp Seeds - omega-3 fatty acids, good source of amino acids, magnesium, and potassium
- Oatmeal – high in fiber and antioxidants
- Pumpkins – beta-carotene
- Quinoa – a complete protein with all 9 amino acids, high in fiber
- Spinach – antioxidants, calcium, vitamin K
- Wild Salmon – omega-3 fatty acids

21 WHAT ARE GOOD CARBS/BAD CARBS?

We love carbs, carbs and more carbs please!!!! Thank God that not all carbs are created equal and we don't have to cut all of them out. But how do you know which ones are good and which ones are bad? Should I do a no-carb, low-carb? With all of the media frenzies surrounding the diet of the week, I would suggest whatever you do, Do Not cut them completely out. It is the body's preferred source of energy. However, if you decide to complete cut them out, do it for a short period of time before you run the risk of getting ketosis. Depending on who you are that may be good for you because it promotes burning fat for fuel, but at the expense of decreased blood sugar levels, depriving your body of carbohydrates, along with constipation, bad breath, weakness, irritability and headaches.

The good news is that carbs aren't all bad even if they existed in very few foods that our ancestors ate. Our ancestors consumed carbohydrates in naturally occurring roots, berries and wild plants foraged throughout their day. Those are good carbohydrates because they are directly from whole foods and are accompanied with fiber and nutrients.

Good carbs are slow releasing energy structures that don't spike your blood sugar levels, leaving you hungry soon after you've eaten them. Bad carbs are refined carbs that are quickly absorbed and released promptly into the bloodstream and rushing through us storing in cells versus being used for energy. Bad carbs rapidly increase our body's insulin levels.

One of the ways carbohydrates are measured to see if they are good or bad is the glycemic index. The glycemic index is what is used to measure how quickly a food substance turns to sugar after eating, basically how it affects our blood glucose levels. Granted this is not a failsafe indicator, but a pretty good measure. There are a few things to make note off.

The glycemic index scale is from 0-100. The scale ranges from low glycemic to high glycemic. When food has a low glycemic index, it provides sustained energy over a period of time, versus a food

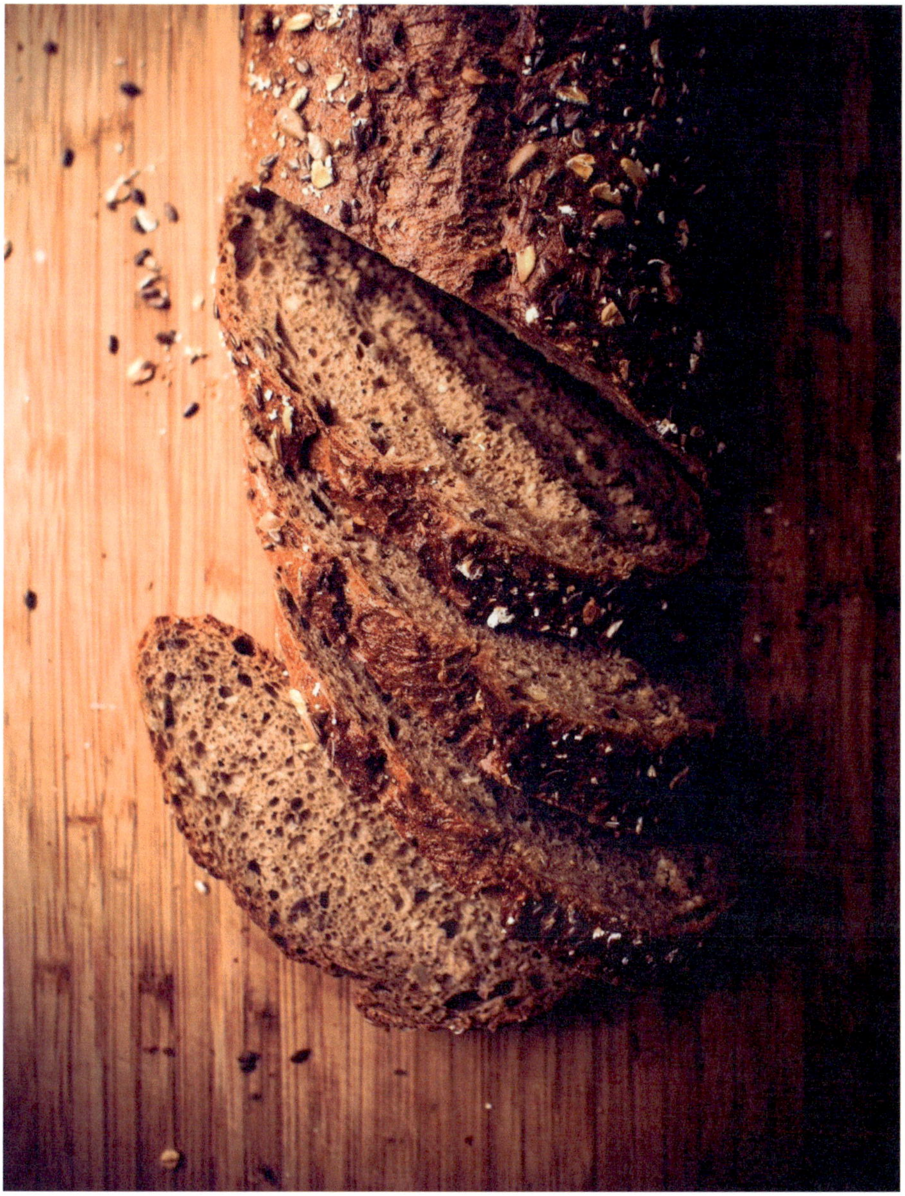

with a high glycemic index which would provide a quick boost of energy, but then you are hungry again that leads to over eating.
Here's an example where the numbers could be confusing and it comes down to making a healthiest decision regardless of the glycemic index. Potato chips glycemic index is 54 and a plain baked potato is 85. Based solely on numbers potato chips would be a

better glycemic choice, however a whole unprocessed potato is the best choice of the two. Carrots and pineapples are between 60 and 80 on the glycemic index, but they are healthier choices than soft drinks and saltine crackers that are also in that index range.

Now that I've explained what good and bad carbohydrates are below are examples of good carbs:

GOOD CARBS

- Old fashioned oatmeal, Barley, buckwheat, bulgur
- Legumes, lentils, peas
- Soybeans
- Grapes, Oranges, Apples, Cherries, Grapefruit, Avocados
- Asparagus, Green Beans
- Yogurt, Milk

BAD CARBS (refined and processed):

- White flour
- White bread, waffles, bagels
- White rice
- Breakfast cereals (most)
- Baked goods
- Snack foods (pretzels/chips)
- Sweets, table sugar
- Sodas

Eating too many highly refined and bad carbohydrate foods leads to obesity, heart disease, and diabetes to name a few. Your diet should consist no more than 50% of calories from carbohydrates. If you want to follow a reduced carb diet then 40% of calories should come from carbohydrates. If you want to take it a step beyond that and try a very low-carb diet stay within 20-30% of your calories coming carbohydrates. If you consume a low-carb diet it will be very important to make sure you are eating adequate amounts of proteins and fats to keep you full and so you are satisfied with each meal.

Benefits of eating low-carb and high protein diets are that you maintain more muscle mass and a healthy metabolism while losing weight. You feel more satisfied with meals because they are higher in protein and fat also causing more calories being burned during the digestion and metabolizing of the food consumed.

21 Cravin'Fit™ HOWS

1 HOW TO THINK Cravin' Fit™

The body does whatever the mind tells it. Your thoughts and beliefs about your abilities shape your outcomes. The actions your body performs are a result of a thought or combination of habits. You cannot completely change your lifestyle until you understand where you currently are and what the new life is all about. Change your thoughts about healthy food and healthy living so that it will manifest into your diet. This process will require some time, so be patient in your quest to learn more about being healthy and what that looks like to you.

Once you have a picture and a vision it starts to build your purpose and you can establish a goal. Whether it's to cut back on the sugar and sodium you consume, increase your vegetable servings, reduce your risk for heart disease, diabetes and cancer, or just understanding what is in the food you are currently consuming. Once your goals are set, get laser focused and devote your daily actions to achieving them.

Some goals may require you to have more discipline to strengthen your self-control. Even if it takes a few dozen tries to reach your goals, each time you try you are getting stronger in your health. Strength is gained by effort and practice. When you attempt something new you must learn first before you are able to master it and succeed. That's how you get strong in the health game. You must train yourself. By changing your thinking to positive thoughts, you will proceed with purpose, think strongly, attempt your goals fearlessly and accomplish with more skills.

Try your very best to block out fear and doubt. Fear that you may not get it right or even eat healthy every single day of your life. The point is to get started right where you are, wherever that may be. Thoughts of fear and doubt can make you feel like this new lifestyle you want to embody is useless and pointless. But I assure you it's not. There is nothing BETTER that you can do for your body than to feed it the best ingredients possible. It prefers it that way.

Ever notice how tired, sluggish and lethargic you feel after eating a large meal, or even something unhealthy. You usually don't feel good. You may even feel guilty. You have satisfied your hunger, but your body suffers. Trying to process all that you fed it, the good, bad and the ugly unnatural foods our bodies were never designed to handle.

Go forward with purpose, energy and believe in your power to be fit. All that you will achieve now are the direct results of your own thoughts. There are sacrifices involved with achievements. The more you sacrifice greater your results will be. Your desire to obtain a healthy life is an achievable aspiration. You receive what you earn; no more and no less.

2 HOW TO GET BACK ON THE FITWAGON?

It's never too late to start. Don't obsess or feel disappointed that you just completely fall off. However when people stop, slip and fall off the bandwagon it is usually because they have gotten bored. You've gotten bored in the health routine and having to monitor and pay special attention to things you didn't think about before. You may have gotten bored with your exercises, your foods, your drinks, your everything!

In order to get the body you want you have to adopt new habits and behaviors. Boredom is often the sign that you need to introduce new things, new foods, new exercises, and new workout spots. If you stop working out it could be because you exceeded your most recent goal and you feel as if you have reached the top. From this point on it is about maintaining your success. So drop in on a dance class to spice up your workouts, go hiking, include swimming, play tennis, racquetball, biking all of these classify as exercise. This also helps take the pressure off of calling it a "workout."

One of the first things you should do if you have fallen off the Cravin'Fit™ food wagon is to up your fruits and vegetable servings. Then reduce the amounts of sugar, salty and processed foods you eat. That's the soda, chips, hot dogs and ice cream. Do you know what they put in hot dogs? Ok I won't tell you, but you might not want to eat them or feed them to your children anymore. Back to the list, then drink more water, eat lean meats, have a few meatless days. Eat less high-fat foods, but include healthy fats, avocado, coconut and olive oils.

It takes 21 days to change or adopt a habit and some studies show that it take up to 66 days, so I call the days after the 21 the commitment phase. This is when the going gets tough and the tough get going!

3 HOW TO SET FITNESS GOALS AND STICK TO IT

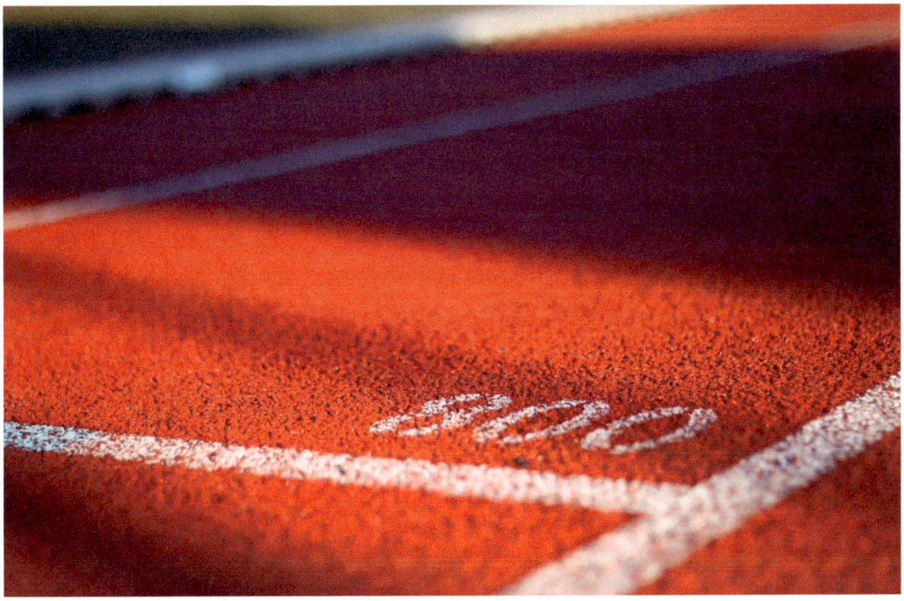

Nine times out of ten you have fitness goals. Whether you actually work towards them, now that's a different story. The most common goals are

- I just want to get fit and workout
- I want to workout more – do you want to be a part of #SquatLife or join CrossFit, a Kickboxing or Barre class?
- I want to try runs and races – mud runs, fun runs, race for the cure, triathlons, marathons, find a cause and run/walk your behind off!
- Get a Six Pack – we all do, but it is achievable if you get your nutrition and physical activity in alignment
- Diet and Lose weight
- I want to challenge myself

Build a positive mentality. A healthy mindset transcends into healthy life. Put gym time in your calendar and schedule it like you would anything else. Don't dread it. Having the ability to be active is a blessing not a curse or a chore. I know personally for me I have to work out no less than three times per week. I even put it in my smart phone to get notifications an hour or two before my sweat session. This is a commitment I make to myself and one you can adopt as your own. Of course it takes time to establish new habits so it's perfectly okay to do once a week for a month, then twice a week for the second month and three times a week in the third month. The point is to get you accustomed to the new lifestyle and also something you can keep going.

If you're the kind of person who struggles with self-motivation, then it might be a good idea to join group classes and bootcamps. Groups are great for morale, support, socializing and you have to keep up with them when exercising.

Strive to be physically active 3 to 4 times per week. Get your heart rate up at least 2 of those times while working out, but 3 is preferable. Individuals who workout and are active lose more weight and keep it off longer than those who don't.

4 HOW MUCH WATER SHOULD I DRINK?

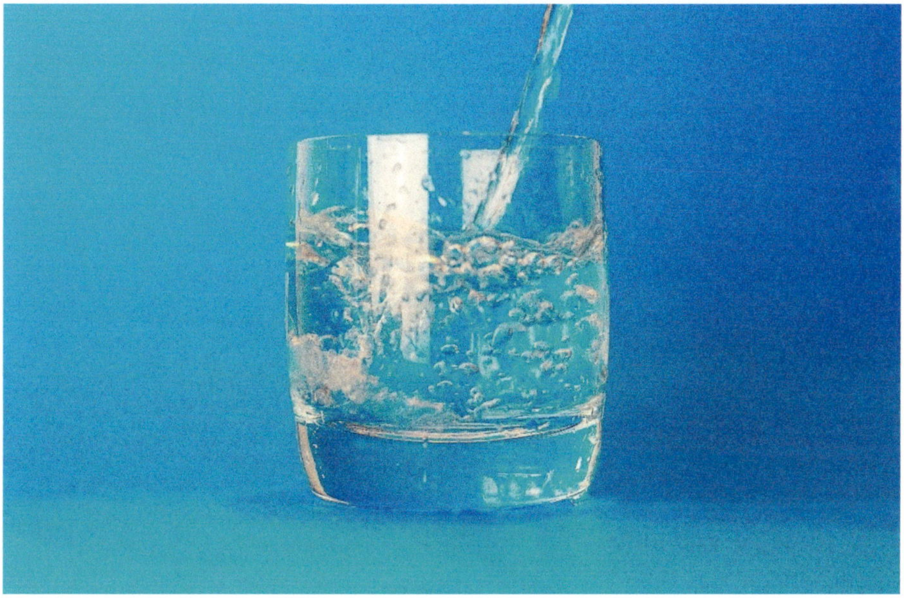

You should drink a lot of water. For some of you, you should drink considerably more than you currently do, but you already knew that. Actually you should consume half your weight in water. The minimum amount of water recommended is 64 ounces per day, hence 8 glasses of water per day. There are 8oz in 1 cup, liquid measurement.

The formula:
Body Weight (lbs) ÷ 2 = Required Water Intake (oz)
If you are 140lbs, divide that by 2 and you need 70 ounces of water per day.

But what if you don't like water? Do you want to live? Okay all jokes aside there are plenty of ways to make water more palatable. There are bazillions of water infusers on the market today. You can infuse your water in a pitcher or a single serve bottle. You can get really creative.

Water Infuser Combinations

- Cucumber, Lime and Mint
- Watermelon and Lime
- Strawberry and Orange
- Grapefruit and Kiwi

5 HOW MUCH SUGAR IS ENOUGH?

Just about everything on the shelves has sugar, added sugar, double sugar and coated with sugar. We are all in our sweet spots. The average person today eats 30 teaspoons of sugar and sweetener per day and some of it is hidden. Would you be surprised if I told you that your healthy low-fat yogurt has more grams of sugar in it than ice cream? If you are surprised, don't be. This is precisely why you must read nutrition labels. This helps you know what is in the item you are about to consume and the quantity of each substance. You cannot leave it to the companies to provide you with 100% healthy options.

As stated above individuals are eating more sugar than the body is designed to handle. The American Heart Association recommends no more than 6 teaspoons (24 grams) a day for women, 9 teaspoons (36 grams) for men and 3 teaspoons (12 grams) for kids. The FDA (Food and Drug Administration) does not require manufacturers to put a Daily Recommended Value for Sugar on their products. So it is up to you to regulate if the product has too much sugar for your consumption or not.

I want to talk briefly about fructose and high-fructose corn syrup (HFCS) and why dieticians and nutritionists like me make such a big stink about not eating it. Fructose does not send signals to the brain indicating we are full. When the brain doesn't receive signals you eat more. Because the signal was never sent this causes you to overeat and potentially gain weight.

Fructose converts to directly fat. Do not pass go, do not collect $200. It isn't the good fat either. When fructose is consumed it is not used right away for energy the way consuming good carbohydrates are. That is why there's such attention on eliminating sodas and some unnatural juices. Fructose is delivered faster. Fructose and HFCS have been known to interfere with fertility, speed up aging and inhibit the immune system

Cravin'Fit Tips:

- Daily limit 6-9 teaspoon of sugar a day

- low-fat might also translate to more sugar, always read the label
- Swap sugar for fats and proteins. Fats and proteins fill you up

Give me some sugar

Below is a list of sugars you may find on ingredient labels and in your food products.

Agave Nectar	Dehydrated Cane Juice	Golden Syrup
Beet Sugar	Dissaccharide	Invert Sugar
Brown Sugar	Ethyl maltol	Lactose
Barley Malt Syrup	Evaporated Cane Juice	Malt syrup
Cane Crystals	Fructose	Maltodextrin
Carob Syrup	Fruit Juice Concentrate	Maltose
Corn Sweetener	Galactose	Monosaccharide
Corn Syrup	Glucose	Monnitol
Crystalline Fructose	High Fructose Corn Syrup	Polysaccharide
Date sugar	Saccharose	Raw sugar
Dextran	Sucrose	Ribose
Dextrin	Sorghum/Sorghum syrup	Rice syrup
Dextrose	Sorbitol	Turbinado
Diastase		

6 HOW MUCH SODIUM DO I NEED?

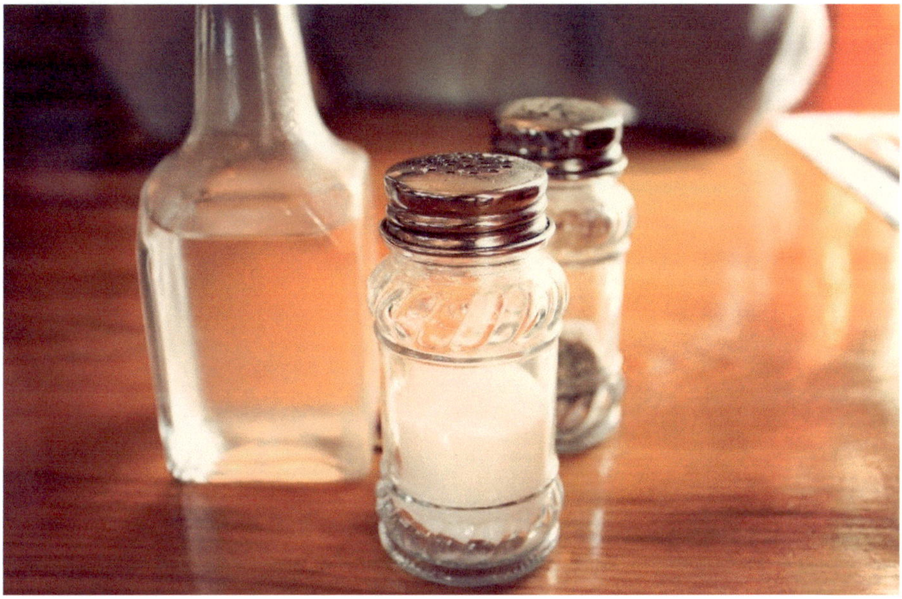

The 2010 Dietary Guidelines recommends 2300mg of sodium per day for the general population. 1500mg for people who are 51 years of age or older, who are African American, and persons with hypertension, diabetes and kidney disease.

A typical meal outside of the home is 2700mg of sodium and not to mention the extra calories. Meals eaten out are generally 200-300 more calories than if you would have prepared it at home yourself.

Do me a favor. The next time you are in the soup aisle at the grocery store, read the sodium count on the Mmm Mmm Good Soup. At the time of publishing, their chicken noodle soup lists 890mg of sodium per serving. At this point we know to check how many servings per container or can in this case. There are 2.5 servings per can. That equates to 2225mg of sodium in one full can. Your entire 2300mg sodium budget is blown on one can of soup. You would need to go salt-less for the rest of the day. #TeamNoSalt

It is important to pay attention to your sodium intake because this raises your blood pressure if you continually eat foods high in sodium. It builds plaque in your veins and arteries causing your heart to work really hard pumping blood through your body. When it is over worked and can't handle the pressure, boom, a heart attack ensues. This doesn't happen in one day, it has been silently building from within. The good news is that healthy eating and exercise can help revert some of the damage caused.

7 HOW MUCH FAT SHOULD I INCLUDE IN MY DIET?

Fat is needed in our daily diets. It is important to include predominately good fats versus the bad fats. Trans-fat are substances you do not want to include in your diet, not even in the tiniest of amounts. Trans-fat is a formed fat when liquid vegetable oil is hydrogenated to make the oil more solid. Manufacturers by law are allowed to label a product free of trans-fat if it has 0.5 grams per serving. The only way to be sure it is absolutely free of trans-fat is to check the list of ingredients on the label. Avoid products containing "shortening" or "partially hydrogenated fats or oils" the main source of trans-fats.

Saturated fats should be avoided because they raise the bad cholesterol, LDL, levels. Fatty meats that are saturated fats increase your risk for heart disease and diabetes. Monounsaturated fats are good fats. This category includes olive oil, avocadoes and most nuts. Polyunsaturated fats are either omega-6 or omega-3. Both are essential for daily life. However the ratios of each are where the difference lies. We should consume considerably more omega-3's than omega-6's which promotes cancer, arthritis and more when there is an imbalance of the two. Popular omega-3 food sources are fatty fish, flaxseed, walnuts and soy.

Healthy fat intake ranges

Children	30-60g
Active Teenagers	40-80g
Women	30-60g
Active Men	40-80g
Athletic Type	80-120g

One of the reasons nutritionists and dieticians recommend the elimination of fried foods is because frying food adds fat. It is also important to note that while olive, coconut and avocado oils are healthy monounsaturated fats, they are still fats. Use these sparingly or measure them. Don't just pour the oil in the pan. One tablespoon of olive oil is 120 calories. So if you have said to yourself, I am eating healthy and exercising but I am not losing any weight, check your preparation methods. This is where the oversight often happens

8 HOW MUCH FIBER SHOULD I CONSUME?

Fiber is the indigestible matter of food. It remains virtually intact from the time it goes into our mouths, through the digestion process and elimination of waste. It ultimately helps waste elimination become a regular and daily occurrence.

If we were to follow the Paleo diet of our ancestors we would roughly consume 47grams of fiber a day. However on average we consume about 10-15 grams a day.

- 38g daily for adult men
- 25g daily for adult women
- 45g daily for active adult men
- 32g daily for active adult women

I want you to reach these goals, but there is no need to make a mad dash to the grocery store to grab the newest flavor of Metamucil ther. When you eat a lot of fried and junk foods there is typically very little fiber in them. Sometimes fiber is added to make up for the lack of nutrition in the food source. I would prefer you get fiber the natural way with fruits, veggies, grains and legumes. Consuming a high-fiber diet helps fight cancer and diseases. The phytonutrients are plant based nutrients present in fiber foods that do most of the fighting.

Cravin'Fit Tip

Black Beans, Pinto Beans and Garbanzo beans are the leading sources of fiber in the bean family.

9 HOW MUCH PROTEIN SHOULD I EAT/DRINK?

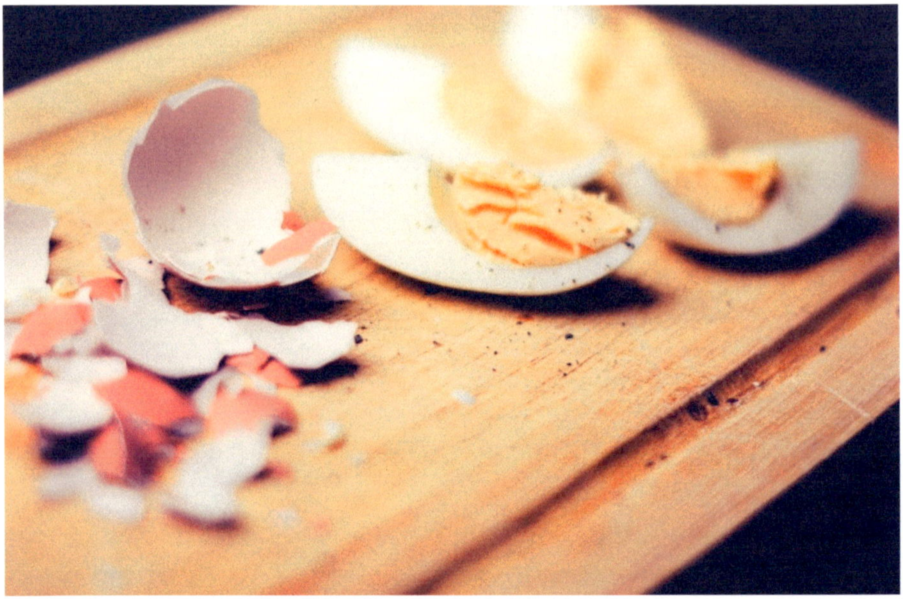

Eating sufficient amounts of protein help preserve muscle mass and helps keep your metabolism high. In general females should eat 3-4oz of protein and males 5-8oz of protein per meal.

The minimum amount of protein you should consume in a day is 0.4 grams per pound of weight. The equation is as follows:

0.4(g of protein) x 140 (lbs) = 56 total grams of protein.

This example is for a 140 pound person who would like to maintain their weight. Athletes and individuals who are highly physically active need more protein to maintain their weight through their strenuous activities.

10 HOW TO EAT THE PERFECT PORTIONS

Eating according to portion sizes is critical to losing and maintaining your weight. It is easy to underestimate portion sizes and calories and boom unknowingly you've eaten more than you needed. How do you know the quantity of foods you eat if you just eye-ball it? I understand some of you may be eyeball professionals, but I am going to implore you to break out the measuring tools. You don't have to go out and buy expensive equipment. You can find many of these items starting at the dollar store, to Wal-Mart, Target or any department store.

Things that no kitchen should be without are measuring spoons, measuring cups and food scale. The food scale is optional but it's pretty tough to measure a ½ cup of chicken breast in the measure cup. It doesn't quite fit. The food scale provides a more accurate calorie count that allows you to take control of your intake.

Let's just say purchasing a scale is not on your radar, well no worries. Nature provided us with the perfect measurement for our individual bodies. It's literally in your hands. Proteins can be measured easily in the palm of your hand at about an inch tall. I discussed the recommended amounts of protein in the previous section so I will skip to carbohydrates and vegetables.

Carbohydrates

The correct amount of good unrefined carbohydrates you should eating are a fist amount. Ball your fist up and this is approximately quantity to eat of brown rice, sweet potatoes and other foods in this category.

Vegetables

There is virtually no limit to this category however it depends on preparation methods; whether or not it is in a sauce, has cheese on it and other toppings we put on vegetables to make them more palatable. The general rule is a double fist of veggies. If you are eating a balanced meal this will be plenty.

Cravin' Fit Tip: Eat on smaller plates, i.e. 8″ plate versus 10″ plate

11 HOW TO MEAL PREP?

Meal planning and prepping can enhance the relationship you have with food. It forces you to give choices more time and attention allowing you to make healthier decisions. Planning in advance can increase your chances for success. It alleviates the "oh what am I going to eat?" "I don't have time cook!" "I want something healthy, nothing is around me...guess I'll go through the drive-thru." Meal prep allows you to be prepared for the week or a few days if you can't plan, or cook for 5-7 days. This is completely customizable to fit you. You can pack all of your snacks for the week and you've technically meal prepped. This is still good and a great first step in the right direction. If you can pack snacks for the week and prep your breakfasts for three days, that's even better. Do what you can when you can.

Determine your meal prep day where you set aside a specific amount of time to get the job done. Taking the time upfront to meal prep saves you calories and headaches during the week when you are trying to find something to eat. The most popular meal prep days are Sunday and Monday, mainly because they are the beginning days of the week. However, you can make any day your meal prep day, or meal prep twice a week. For instance Sunday and Wednesday could be your days or Monday and Thursday.

Next, purchase BPA-free Tupperware sets, or use glass. Glass sets cost a tad bit more, but they are stain resistant when you have spaghetti with zucchini or spaghetti squash noodles. If you are anything like me, I don't like my food touching so I have containers with three separate compartments.

Decide what you will eat for the week, make a grocery list and don't pick up any junk food when you at the grocery store. Once you get home, wash and cut fruits and veggies that you will use for your meals, snacks, salads, juice and smoothies. Then make your marinade and marinate any meat or tofu if your recipe calls for it. Cook your meals accordingly. Then when you items are finished, break out your measuring utensils or food scale and divide your food in containers until it's all gone.

Cravin'Fit Tips:

- Bag smoothie or juice ingredients in Ziploc bags. Label the bags the day of use with a permanent marker.
- When making salads, try assembling your salads in a Mason Jar. Putting the wet ingredients at the bottom, the dressing, tomatoes, avocadoes then layer with sturdier ingredients on top, bell peppers, cucumbers, celery, then your kale, spinach, or romaine lettuce. If you don't have Mason jars, use large Tupperware bowls and assemble the same way.
- Boiling eggs in a batch is a real life saver when you are rushing in the morning, just grab an egg and go.
- Stick to the schedule and have yourself a cheat meal or cheat day. I don't want you to be totally restricted, but keep in mind some of the things I strongly suggest avoiding like trans-fat and high fructose corn syrup.

12 HOW TO EAT HEALTHY ON A BUDGET

- Rule number 1: Don't buy high-fat, high calorie foods! If you have them in the house, fridge or pantry you will eat them. They might even call out your name, subconsciously at least.
- Shop the weekly circular sales paper from the grocery stores that come in the mail then plan your meals around that
- Buy frozen vegetables when they are on sale
- Buy organic when your wallet allows and when organic items are on sale.
- Buy produce that's in season which is also a good way to keep selections diverse and ensure you are eating a variety of foods.
- Use coupons, buy the Sunday paper and get your scissors out
- Shop the perimeter of the grocery store aisle
- Shop Asian and ethnic grocery stores and markets. Also a great place to get fresh spices and uncommon ingredients.
- Go to the farmers market at the end of the day and play, let's make a deal, not literally the game, but it is a good time to get reduced prices...they don't really want to go back home with the items

13 HOW TO BOOST YOUR METABOLISM?

- Exercise boosts your metabolism. Exercise is so good for you that it increases your metabolic rate for hours after you have worked out. Which essentially burns more fat, post workout.
- Don't skip breakfast. Breakfast jumpstarts your metabolism and stabilizes blood sugar levels, so that you don't overeat throughout the day.
- Drinking water (especially cold) – cold water forces the body to use more energy to warm the cold water up to your normal body temperature.
- Gain lean muscle mass. Lean muscles increase your metabolism. Yes Yes, I know. You only want to do cardio and don't want muscles, but want to lose weight. How else are you going to burn more fat? The more muscle you have the more fat you burn. You must include strength training in your exercise routines. You don't need to do this every day, but it definitely needs to be a regular part of your routine, if you are physically able.
- Sauna – really good for people who have disabilities who cannot physically workout. This is not to completely exclude working out for physically capable beings it is another option to explore. Sauna heat causes you to sweat and therefore raises your metabolic rate and burn more calories.
- Eat protein– digestion is a laborious process, it takes work to turn steak into nutrients that the body can use for energy.
- Eat Frequently
- Drink Green Tea

It is a great idea to incorporate high intensity interval training. This is where you do a set of cardio exercises for a predetermined time period, take a quick recovery break and do it again. Since my days as a track athlete I have long known the benefits of interval training. At that time I wasn't quite worried about the increased fat burn as a result of interval training. I was more focused on the endurance, stamina and speed it provided me in my sprints.

14 HOW TO CONTROL SWEET CRAVINGS?

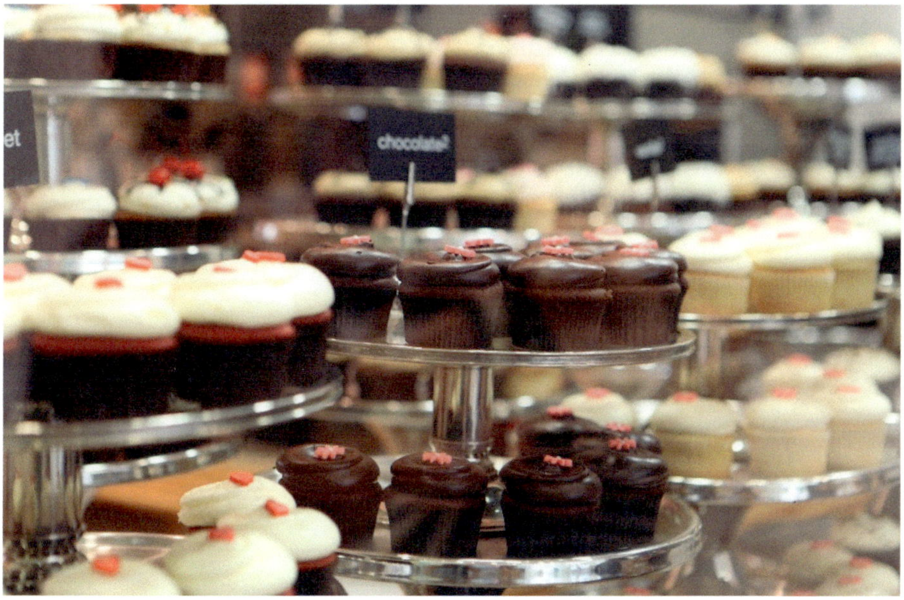

How do we satisfy a sweet tooth? Doughnuts and honey buns for breakfast. Cupcake after lunch, a Twix bar at 3 o'clock, ice cream after dinner we are just swimming in a sea of sugar. Please enjoy and indulge in your sweet tooth from time to time. After all you are human. Allow yourself a treat, but make it special. Don't completely ban sweets that will just make you want them more but try the following methods more often than giving in to temptation.

- Hurry and grab the sweetest fruit close to you, watermelon, cherries, mangos, pineapples...the list continues.
- Chew sugar-free gum, aspartame free.
- Instead of milk chocolate switch to dark chocolate. Just melt a little bit of dark chocolate in a bowl with a teaspoon or so of coconut oil and dip banana, apple slices or strawberries in them.
- Eat low, reduced or no added sugar cinnamon applesauce.
- You can also try brushing your teeth. Usually when you brush your teeth you don't want to eat anything immediately

after it. Food doesn't taste the same if you eat it right after you've freshly brushed your teeth.

- Use stevia in recipes to reduce your sugar intake, as well as using it in tea, coffee etc. Stevia is an herb used as sweetener.
- Also before you indulge, try to engage in an activity to take your mind off of it pick up a book or magazine.
- Go visit a coworker in the next cubicle, grab a family member to go on a quick walk, call that person you've been meaning to catch up with.

15 HOW TO FIND GOOD SUPPLEMENTS?

Supplements are designed to help you reach your goals quicker. You should always take a multi-vitamin. The second supplement I recommend is EPA/DHA, fish oil, for women get 500-1000mg and men 1000-2000mg. Another way to get more omega-3 fatty acids are by adding flaxseed to cereal, oatmeal, chia pudding and smoothies.

Here is how you know if you are taking good quality supplements or not, perform this test:

Drop the supplement pill in a 4-6oz glass of vinegar warmed to about 98 degrees. Allow 45minutes to an hour for the results. The test is done using vinegar because it most closely mimics our stomach acids.

- If the pill breaks all the way down and dissolves completely it is a good supplement and your body will likely absorb it quickly and efficiently.
- If it never breaks down it has binders in it
- If it is chalky on the top then it has fillers, like sand and silicone

When you take supplements that aren't good quality, the residue you see as a result of the test pass through the body unused. Some manufactures use binders and fillers such as sawdust and sand. That's crazy right? Fillers are often added to make production faster, pills more appealing or easier to swallow. You think you are taking supplements to put good substances in you, when really you are ingesting foreign materials your body was never designed to handle.

Cravin'Fit Tips:

- Vitamins are no substitute for a healthy diet.
- Creatine is best used for activities like bench pressing, short bursts of energy like sprints and is more beneficial for individuals who perform day long trainings.
- CLA (conjugated linoleic acid) enhances weight loss and

helps build lean muscle

- Protein powder - you can get adequate amounts from your daily diet. However, I understand if you had a hard late night workout and then you drink a protein shake after versus, eating a full meal then going to bed without fully digesting that high protein meal. The shake allows for easier digestion, and an lighter stomach feel before bed.

16 HOW TO BURN MORE CALORIES?

Interval training is where you do periods of high intensity, combined with periods of low intensity. An Australian study in the International Journal of Obesity found young women who alternated between 8 seconds of high-intensity and 12 seconds of low-intensity exercise for just 20 minutes three times a week burned more fat than did steady-state exercisers who logged twice as much time breaking a sweat.

Build your endurance so you can get stronger in your interval training. You build endurance through aerobic exercises, running, swimming or biking where you are going at a steady pace for longer periods of time. You can also build endurance through other aerobic exercises such as dancing, who hasn't heard of Zumba?

Give 100% more in your workouts. We've all been there right, you do just enough to get by and no more. When we are no longer killing our workouts it is a sign to turn it up a notch, put more into it and you get more out. More equals more, do more, get more.

Add leg weights or body weighted vest. This will provide the extra resistance you need forcing your body to do more work because of the added weight. Lift heavier weights. This is a sure fire way to burn more calories, because you are working harder to control the resistance through the exercises. Besides, lifting heavier weights builds more muscles which in turns burns more calories and fat.

Grab a friend, while it's not proven that you will burn more calories, but you might go longer and harder if you have someone else working out with you to keep you accountable.

Cravin'Fit Tip

1. Purchase a heart rate monitor, then you will know when you are in your target heart rate zone
2. Purchase a pedometer because more steps are better than no steps.

17 HOW TO GAIN MORE MUSCLE AND NOT BECOME A BODYBUILDER?

Muscle facts, one pound of muscle tissue burns between 35 and 50 calories per day. More muscle mass equals greater fat burning rates. It is totally acceptable to have a love for cardio. There is a point in cardio where you are burning muscle and that is why it is important to include strength training in your exercise routine.

Strength training is here to stay, according to the annual survey by the American College of Sports Medicine. It ranks number 2, up from number 6 in 2007 according to the poll of 2,620 fitness professionals, including certified trainers and exercise physiologists.

Women are notorious for not wanting to lift weight because they will look bulky. Honestly honey, you really aren't going to put in that much work to look even remotely close to Arnold Schwarzenegger, nor do you have enough testosterone to achieve that. However, I understand not everyone likes the look of muscles or being really defined. Sometimes you just have to accept your genes, be healthy and move on.

For instance Serena Williams, she is not designed to be a size zero. Even if she tried to lose weight and not saying she is. She is very fit, has an athletic build and that is her body shape for life. Introducing #ThickFit where women are embracing their curves and being the healthiest they can possibly be at their size.

If you want to maintain your muscles, do light to medium weights with high reps. If you want to get stronger and build muscles go heavier on the weights. Then once you have reached your ideal shape, go back down to light to medium weights or use your own body weight.

Make sure to include rest days. Do not strength train the same muscle group every day, especially if you used heavy weights and are sore. We want to prevent injury as much as possible. Include stretches, a warm up or warm up sets in your routine. If you have any time left at the end of your workout do 5 minutes of cool down.

Always practice proper form in all moves, squat, lunge, deadlifts. Don't move fast through the moves. If you are interested in or perform cross-fit this is extremely important to pay attention to your form. Too hard and too fast can land you on your butt quicker than how you got started.

Cravin'Fit Tips:

- In the beginning it is important to learn to perform the exercises correctly
- Strength train 2-3 times per week.
- Beginners: do one set of 12-15 repetitions per exercise. Then throughout the weeks increase the number of sets you perform.
- Try not to do too much too soon.
- Try muscle groups, like legs, have a leg day, or upper body, or chest and shoulders and back or abdominals and lower back.

A total body workout should include 10 large muscle groups. *Example of total body workout:*

- leg press or squats
- dead lifts or leg curls
- knee extensions (if your knees allow this)
- bench press
- horizontal rows, crunches
- lateral pull-downs, shoulder press, arm curls, tricep extensions and calf raises.

You can also perform pyramids once you are comfortable with the moves.

- Perform 4-6 repetitions with a lower weight or body weight
- Increase your next set to 8-10 repetitions with heavier weights
- Increase your 3rd set to 12-15 with the heaviest weight

18 HOW TO EAT 6 TIMES A DAY, OR CLOSE TO IT

Six times per day may be a lot for some people. However I am not suggesting six full course meals. I suggest three square meals and three snacks. Think of it as you are nourishing your body six times per day. I understand this may require reprogramming and pre-planning. It is certainly worth the effort you put in if you take advantage of meal prepping.

Eating less frequent slows your metabolism and your body holds onto the extra weight because it doesn't know the next time it will be nourished. It uses the stored fat for energy when you don't eat. Eating 1-2 times per day thwarts any efforts you have of losing weight or living healthy the natural way. By eating more frequent meals it makes it easier to maintain your ideal weight.

You can eat protein shake or bar for one of those meals, a smoothie or a juice for the other, and fruit for the third snack. It is always a good idea to eat a few grams of protein in your snacks. When the body goes without protein for four hours plus, the body breaks down muscle tissue to use. We don't want that to happen especially after we spent time building muscles.

Cravin'Fit Tip

Try not to load up on carbohydrates before bed. I know you may have heard this a million times. The reason is as explained earlier carbohydrates primary purpose is to be used immediately for energy and you don't need that much energy to sleep. So whatever you don't burn off before bed gets stored as fat. The recommendation is to eat carbs earlier in your day and very few at night. Dinner should consist of protein, low fat and a vegetable. However if you are running a marathon the next day it's okay to increase your carb intake at dinner.

19 HOW TO PLOW THROUGH A PLATEAU

Plateaus are a part of the game. The best thing for a plateau is a switch up. You can't do the same ole same ole anymore. Your body has gotten accustomed to the food and exercises. Find something new. Never get bored, the possibilities are endless.

Make sure you are getting plenty of rest, keep your stress levels down if at all possible. Also, you may have relaxed a bit in your food preparation methods and possibly underestimated portions and oils used. Check back in with your serving sizes, exercise portion control and continue to read food labels and keep your food journal up to date. At this point you should be in the habit of reading every food label of the products you purchase and eat. Don't make a purchase without reading the label and ingredient list.

20 HOW TO STOP EATING WHEN I'M FULL

We eat with our eyes first. Our eyes are often bigger than our stomachs. Even thinking about certain foods makes our mouth water. We want a food and want to get our justly fill. It takes approximately twenty minutes for your stomach to send the message to your brain that you are full. I know we've all been there, when we were just beyond starving and scarfed down the food in front of us. The action was probably one chomp short of swallowing our food whole. I encourage you to slow down while eating and chew your food completely before adding another spoonful in your mouth. When you properly chew your food before swallowing, you are releasing nutrients that your body can digest easier. The digestion process begins in the mouth and helps eliminate waste better. Take the time to savor and enjoy your meal, away from distractions or activities where the focus isn't on your current food consumption.

Fiber is perfect to keep you full as well as fat and protein to help you feel satiated. There are a few things you can do to recognize when you have reached the limit. One is you must get more in tune with what your body signals. If you begin to feel bloating or stretching to accommodate more food, then you should stop. Also when you eat more food than what your healthy portion size should be, it slows your metabolism.

Cravin'Fit Tips:

- Drink an 8oz glass of water before a meal
- Eat a small piece of fruit, an apple, before a meal
- Eat1 cup of tomato or vegetable broth based soup before a meal

21 HOW TO CHOOSE THE RIGHT FOODS WHEN EATING OUT

Let's face it going out to eat is a part of life, community and being social. However you can still make good choices while out having fun and enjoying healthy light fare. Below are simple tips to not break the calorie budget.

- Choose lean protein and vegetables
- Salad - don't top it with fried foods like chicken, that's an oxymoron
- Skip the fried food
- Choose low-fat, fat-free or low sodium dressing, oil and vinegar works as well
- Get dressing, sauces, syrup on the side
- Have the waiter remove the bread or not bring any out
- Swap white potatoes for sweet potatoes
- Swap white rice for wild or brown rice or quinoa if they have it
- Ask questions about preparation methods, butter, oils, etc and make requests to eliminate or go light on those items
- If you get dessert, share it, take half home or get 3 bites and have the waiter remove it
- Pizza – forgo the double stuffed crust and add a few more veggies than you normally would. Also choose a whole grain crust wherever available. Thin crust pizzas save you calories as well over the traditional deep dish or regular style.

21 Cravin'Fit™ MEALS

MORE THAN CHICKEN BREAST, STEAMED BROCCOLI, BROWN RICE AND SWEET POTATOES

I know you've seen this before...If you want to be healthy you need to only eat baked chicken breast, steamed broccoli, brown rice and baked sweet potatoes. Well this is fine if this is all you know in the beginning and if it helps get you started quicker then BOOM. Let's season this chicken and get started. In this section of the book I hope to provide you with meals on meals on meals so that you don't have to eat the same thing all the time.

Again, this is a healthy lifestyle, not an 100% hands-off type of meal deal. You want a cookie or a sweet treat that seems to not be a part of healthy eating. I just want you to be aware of what you are eating, enjoy your food and then also work in your favorite foods from time to time. It's alright to indulge on occasion, but if you do this every day then it is not an indulgence, it becomes negligence.

SELF-DISCIPLINE

The ability to make yourself do, what you should do, when you should do it, whether you feel it or not.

21 Cravin'Fit BREAKFASTS

KEY:

DF – diabetic friendly	**GF** – gluten-free
LC – low carb	**HP** – high protein
P – paleo	**VE** – vegan
VG – vegetarian	

Amelia's Muesli - diabetic friendly, gluten-free, vegetarian

¾ cup toasted oats
1 medium apple, chopped
⅛ tsp ground cinnamon
¾ cup unsweetened soy or almond milk
1 tsp unsweetened shredded coconut or handful of coconut flakes
2 tbsp walnuts, chopped
2 tsp dried cranberries

1. *How to Roast Oats:* take 4 cups of old-fashioned rolled oats and spread out on unsprayed baking sheet. Bake in oven at 250°F for 45minutes until golden brown. Cool before storing in a container
2. Place oats and walnuts in a cereal bowl. Add remaining ingredients, stir and enjoy.

Yield 1 serving; 1⅔ cup; 469 calories, 17g protein, 71mg sodium

Cravin'Fit Tip: eat one cup to cut calories and stay around 300

Bananaloupe Smoothie - paleo

2 ripe bananas
½ ripe cantaloupe, cut into chunks, remove the rinds
¼ cup unsweetened almond milk, or coconut milk
1 cup of ice

1. Blend first 3 ingredients until smooth
2. Add ice and blend to desired consistency

Yield 2 servings

Shrimp Tomata Fritatta - low carb, gluten-free

2 whole eggs
2 tsp olive oil
¼ cup grated, reduced-fat cheddar cheese
1 medium red bell pepper, sliced (2 cups)
½ pound cooked shrimp, cut in half
Salt & freshly ground pepper
6 egg whites
1 medium tomato, sliced

1. Preheat the oven to 400°F. Lightly beat the whole eggs and egg whites together in a medium bowl, season with salt and pepper to taste

2. Heat oil in a medium nonstick skillet over medium heat. Add the pepper and sauté for 3 minutes. Add the shrimp and pour the egg mixture into the pan, swirl mixture in the pan to cover peppers. Allow to set for 1 minute.
3. Place the tomato slices on top and sprinkle with the cheese
4. Place in the oven for 5 minutes or until the eggs are set to the desired consistency. Cut into 2 and serve or save for meal prep

Yield 2 servings

Peaches & Cream Oat Crunch – low sugar

1 medium peach, chopped and thoroughly washed (use a fruit and vegetable spray)
¼ cup almond milk, or preferred non-dairy milk
½ cup dry steel-cut oats
1 cup water
Cinnamon to taste
¼ cup chopped pecans
½ tsp sea salt (optional especially if you are doing a no-salt diet)

1. Mix oats, water and salt in a saucepan; cover and soak overnight
2. In the morning heat oats over medium heat until creamy, 5-10 minutes
3. Remove from heat, stir in peaches, almond milk, cinnamon and pecans
4. Pour into a bowl to enjoy or mason jar to enjoy on your way to work

Yield 1, Serving size 1 cup; 312 calories, 42g carbohydrates, 8g of protein, 14g fat, 12g fiber, sugars 8g

Avocado Egg Salad - gluten-free

7 hard boiled eggs, peeled and cooled
1 avocado, peeled, pitted and cut into 1" pieces
2 tbsp plain Greek low-fat yogurt, gluten free
2 tbsp lemon juice
1 green onion, finely chopped
1 celery stalk, finely chopped
1 tsp paprika
½ tsp salt
½ tsp pepper

1. Separate the yolks and the egg whites. Set aside 3 yolks for separate use.

2. Dice the egg whites
3. In a large bowl, combine the avocado, 4 egg yolks and yogurt. Mash until the mixture is creamy and smooth.
4. Mix in the lemon juice, onion, celery, paprika, salt and pepper
5. Gently add the chopped egg whites and combine.
6. Serve on roll up in a gluten-free tortilla, or toast, English muffin, collard leaf
7. refrigerate leftovers

Yield 6

Cravin'Fit Addition: eat with a banana or grapefruit

Bulgar Butt – low sodium

3 cups presoaked bulgur
2 tbsp creamy almond butter
¼ tsp ground cinnamon
1 cup chopped peeled tart-sweet apple
¼ cup plain reduced-fat Greek yogurt
2 ounces feta or blue cheese, crumbled
2 tbsp thinly sliced almonds, toasted
2 tsp honey

- Combine bulgur, almond butter, and cinnamon, stirring well. Add apple; toss. Combine yogurt and goat cheese, stirring until smooth. Divide bulgur mixture among 4 bowls; top evenly with yogurt mixture. Sprinkle with almonds, and drizzle with honey.

Yield 4, serving size: approx 1 cup bulgur; 298 calories, 41g carbohydrates, 14g protein, fat 10.5g, 8g fiber, 121mg sodium, 12g sugar

Cravin'Fit Tip: for variation use pumpkin pie spice in place of cinnamon and replace apple with roasted sweet potato, chopped

Chocolate Chip Banana Muffins - gluten-free, oil-free, sugar free

2 eggs
2 ripe bananas
¼ cup honey
1 cup Greek yogurt
2 cups gluten-free rolled oats
1½ tsp baking powder
½ tsp. baking soda
½ cup mini dark chocolate chips

1. Preheat oven to 375°
2. Mix wet ingredients separate from dry ingredients
3. Blend all wet and dry ingredients (excluding chocolate chips) together in a food processor until smooth. Add chocolate chips and stir to distribute
4. Pour or scoop mixture into muffin tins, spray tins with cooking spray if you aren't using cupcake/silicone liners. Sprinkle a few chocolate chips on the top (optional) Bake for 25-30 minutes until tops of muffins are set

Yields 12

Sweet Potato Bread – gluten-free, oil free

1 ½ cups of oat flour
2 tbsp brown sugar, or blend
¼ cup applesauce
1 tsp vanilla
1 tsp baking powder
½ tsp nutmeg
⅓ stevia or other granulated sugar
1 cup mashed sweet potato
⅓ cup egg whites
1 tsp baking soda
1 tsp cinnamon
¼ tsp salt
⅓ cup chopped pecans (optional)

1. Preheat oven to 350°F
2. Combine all ingredients in a large bowl, stirring in pecans last if using. Transfer to a loaf pan or 2 smaller ones sprayed with cooking spray. Top with additional pecans
3. Bake approximately 35 minutes for one loaf pan or 25 minutes for the 2 smaller ones, do the toothpick test. If the top begins to burn a little cover the top with aluminum foil

Yield 10 slices, serving size 1 slice; 96 calories, 14g carbohydrates, 4g protein, 3g fat

Tropical Mango Smoothie Bowl - low-fat, gluten-free, vegetarian

1 cup frozen mango
½ cup frozen pineapple chunks
⅓ cup low-fat plain Greek yogurt
⅓ cup coconut water
¼ tsp turmeric

Toppings
2 tsp hemp or chia seeds
2 tbsp toasted coconut or coconut flakes
¼ cup blueberries

1. Blend first 5 ingredients until smooth. Pour into a bowl
2. Top with hemp or chia seeds, coconut flakes and blueberries

Yield 1

Cravin'Fit Tip: for more protein add a half scoop of favorite vanilla protein powder

Sweet Pork Sausage with Potato Hash & Sautéed Kale - paleo

2 lbs ground pork (80% lean 20% fat)
2 tbsp pure maple syrup
1 tbsp kosher salt
1 tsp freshly ground pepper
2 tsp fresh sage; minced
1 tsp fresh thyme; minced
½ tsp fresh rosemary; minced
½ tsp ancho chile powder
2 tbsp oil of choice

1. In a large bowl, mix all the ingredients together except the oil. Don't over mix
2. With your hands form 16 rounds, like small patties, about ¾" high
3. Melt oil in cast iron or large skillet pan over medium heat. Cook 8 at a time 4minutes per side, remove to a paper towel lined plate, then cook the remaining 8

Yield 16

Sweet Potato Hash

2 large sweet potatoes, washed, peeled and shredded

In a medium skillet heat 2 tbsp oil of choice add sweet potatoes and cook until tender 6-8minutes, stirring often

Sautéed Kale

½ cup low-sodium vegetable broth
½ yellow onion
Salt and pepper to taste
2 cups of kale

- In a medium pan add broth, onions and kale, cook on medium high heat for 5-7minutes or until kale is wilted and tender

Very Velma Vanilla Smoothie Bowl – gluten-free

7 whole frozen strawberries
½ cup ice, crushed
¼ tsp vanilla extract
2 dates, chopped and pitted
3 tbsp rolled oats, gluten free
⅓ cup coconut milk

Toppings
2 strawberries
½ small banana sliced
¼ cup granola

1. Blend ingredients until smooth. Pour into a bowl and top with toppings.

Yield 1

Steak and Eggs Florentine – paleo, high protein

4 - 4oz lean beef tenderloin steaks about 1 ½ inches thick
8 eggs, egg whites or egg substitutes
2 cups spinach
4 garlic cloves, peeled
4 lemon wedges
¼ cup low-fat feta cheese
1 ½ tbsp olive oil
2 ½ tsp fresh rosemary, chopped
1 small roma tomato, diced

1. Preheat grill or use a cast iron grill pan to medium-high heat
2. Put 1 tbsp olive oil, rosemary, and garlic in a food processor, pulse and process until it becomes a paste
3. Season steaks with salt and pepper then spread the paste mixture on both sides of the steak
4. Grill or cook 5 minutes per side or until desired doneness
5. Heat ½ tbsp olive oil medium pan over medium-high heat and sauté until just wilted transfer to plate, top with tomatoes and feta (split between 4 servings)
6. Spray the same medium pan with cooking spray and

scramble the eggs over medium-high heat

7. When the eggs are done top each spinach batch with the eggs alongside the steak

Yields 4

Apple Baked Oats - diabetic friendly, gluten-free, vegetarian

¾ cup apple, chopped
1½ cup unsweetened almond/soymilk
½ tsp salt
1 tbsp unsweetened shredded coconut
1½ cup old-fashioned rolled oats
½ tsp vanilla extract
½ tsp ground cinnamon
¼ cup walnuts, chopped

- Preheat oven to 350°F Spread the apple on the bottom of the 8-inch square baking dish. Distribute the oats evenly over the apples. In a medium bowl briefly whisk the milk, vanilla, salt and cinnamon together. Pour slowly over the apples and oats. Sprinkle the coconut and walnuts on top. Bake for 45minutes until golden brown

Yield 8 servings

Stir-Fry Bacon – gluten-free, paleo

4 bacon strips, low sodium and nitrate free
1 head broccoli, chopped
1 cup white mushrooms, sliced
1 red bell pepper, sliced
2 cups cabbage, shredded
Salt and pepper to taste

1. Heat a heavy skillet over medium heat
2. Cook the bacon until crispy
3. Add the broccoli, bell pepper, mushrooms and cabbage
4. Continue to stir-fry vegetables until soft, then season with salt and pepper

Yield 2 servings

Cravin'Fit Addition: enjoy alongside 2 eggs prepared your favorite way

Don't Take Me for Granate Smoothie – paleo, vegetarian

1 cup blueberries
½ cup unsweetened almond milk
1 tbsp honey
1 large apple, cored, and chopped
½ cup pomegranate juice (unsweet)
1 cup of ice

1. Blend all ingredients except the ice until smooth
2. Add ice and blend to desired consistency

Yield 2 servings

Don't Come Moroccan Eggs - low-carb

1 tbsp olive oil
½ tsp ground cumin
¼ cup canned diced tomatoes
½ tsp minced garlic or 1 clove garlic, crushed
¼ cup chopped onion
1 tbsp tapenade
3 eggs
2 tbsp fresh cilantro, chopped

1. In a skillet, heat the olive oil over high heat, sauté the onion and garlic until the onion is translucent, then add the tapenade and tomatoes to stir.
2. Whisk the eggs with the cumin, pour eggs into the vegetable scramble. Scramble until mostly set, then add cilantro and continue to scramble until done. Salt & pepper to taste, and serve

Yield: 1 serving; 11g carbohydrates, 18g protein, 1g Fiber

Cravin'Fit Tip: Goes good with Sweet Pork Sausage on page 76, or low sodium nitrate-free turkey sausage or turkey bacon and 1 cup of berries

Blueberry Nana Oatmeal Smoothie - gluten-free

¾ cup fresh or frozen blueberries, organic if possible
½ cup gluten-free rolled oats
1 banana; frozen
4-5 cubes of ice, if using fresh berries
1 cup soy or almond milk
1 tsp honey (optional)

1. Place oats in blender and blend for 1-2 minutes until they are finely ground into a powder
2. add the rest of the ingredients, blend and enjoy.

Zucchini & Sausage casserole – gluten free

1 lb mild pork sausage, gluten free, or preferred sausage
1¼ cups parmesan cheese, grated, fresh or gluten-free
3 medium zucchini, sliced into ½" rounds
½ tsp salt
1 tsp mint, dried
½ tsp basil
1 cup whole milk
½ tsp pepper, freshly ground
½ tsp dried oregano
2 large eggs, beaten
1 small onion, sliced

1. In a large skillet, brown sausage, drain fat from skillet, set sausage aside
2. Grease a 4 qt slow cooker with nonstick spray. In a large bowl whisk together the parmesan cheese, salt, pepper, and mint, oregano and basil. In another bowl whisk together the eggs and milk.
3. Place ⅓ of the zucchini over the bottom of the slow cooker. Add ⅓ sliced onions over the zucchini. Add ⅓ sausage over the onions. Add ⅓ of milk/egg mixture over the sausage. Lastly add ⅓ parmesan cheese mixture over everything. (Repeat layering until you run out, about 2 times)
4. Cover, vent lid with a skewer or chopstick and cook on low for 6 hours or on high for 3 hours. Cut into squares and serve

Yield 6

Grape-Ape Strawberry Muffins - vegan, vegetarian

2 ripe bananas
Half an apple
¼ cup canola oil
1 tsp baking soda
1 cup strawberries (about 12)
½ cup red grapes (12 to 15)
1½ cups whole wheat flour
1 tsp salt

1. Preheat oven to 350 degrees.
2. Peel the bananas, place them in a medium bowl, and mash with a fork.
3. Chop the strawberries, apple, and grapes until minced, and add those to the bowl.
4. Stir in the oil. Add the flour, baking soda, and salt. Put paper or silicone muffin cups in a muffin pan, and pour in the

batter, filling each cup about three-quarters full (makes 15 muffins).

5. Bake for about 18 to 20 minutes or until a toothpick inserted comes out clean.
6. Allow muffins to cool on a rack, and enjoy!

Yield 15, 100 calories; 15.3g carbohydrates, 1.5g protein, 3.8g fat, 240mg sodium, 3.6g sugar

Cravin'Fit Addition: enjoy with ½ tbsp of your favorite nut butter, an additional 90-110 calories

Cinnamon Roll Smoothie - vegan

1 frozen banana, cut into four pieces
½ tsp ground cinnamon
½ tsp pure maple syrup
1 cup unsweetened almond milk
¼ tsp vanilla extract
Cinnamon stick, for garnish

1. Combine all ingredients in a blender. Blend until smooth, and add more almond milk if necessary.
2. Pour into a tall glass, add the cinnamon stick for garnish, and enjoy.

Yield 1, calories 157; 3.7g fat, protein 2.3g, 172mg sodium

Cravin'Fit Tip: for more protein add our favorite vanilla or plain protein powder

Black Bean Avocado Toast - vegetarian

1 slice of Ezekiel, whole grain or wheat, toasted
⅓ cup black beans, drained, rinsed and mashed
⅓ cup ripe avocado, mashed
Black pepper
Lemon to squeeze on top

1. Mash black beans with a fork in a small bowl
2. Mash avocado with fork in a small bowl
3. Toast bread and spread mashed beans on top, then add mashed avocadoes on top, squeeze lemon on top toast, season with pepper
4. Enjoy with grapefruit and orange slices (vegetarian)

Cravin'Fit Addition: Feel free to add 1 fried whole egg on top or, egg white

21 Cravin'Fit LUNCHES

KEY:

DF – diabetic friendly
LC – low carb
P – paleo
VG – vegetarian
GF – gluten-free
HP – high protein
VE – vegan

Burrito Bowl - vegetarian

1 cup uncooked rice
1 cup salsa, homemade or store-bought
3 cups chopped Romaine lettuce
1 15.25oz can whole kernel corn, drained
1 15oz black beans, drained and rinsed
2 Roma tomatoes, diced
1 avocado, halved, seeded, peeled and diced
2 tbsp chopped fresh cilantro leaves

1. To make the chipotle cream sauce, whisk together sour cream, chipotle paste, garlic, lime juice and salt; set aside.
2. In a large saucepan of 1½ cups water, cook rice according to package instructions; let cool and stir in salsa; set aside.
3. To assemble the bowls, divide rice mixture into serving bowls; top with lettuce, corn, black beans, tomatoes, avocado and cilantro.
4. Serve immediately, drizzled with chipotle cream sauce.
5. Roasted Red Pepper Dressing

Chili Dippin Crudités - gluten-free

½ lb ground beef, chicken or turkey
1 medium onion, chopped
2 cloves garlic, chopped
1 tbsp extra virgin olive oil
¼ tsp ground pepper
4 tsp chili powder (gluten-free)
½ cup flat gluten-free beer
1 13oz can red kidney beans; drained and rinsed
Low fat Cheddar cheese, shredded (optional)
2 jalapeño peppers, cored, seeded, and chopped (use 1 for less heat)

1. Sauté the meat with onion, peppers and garlic in a large skillet, stirring and crumbling meat with a wooden or plastic spoon
2. When the vegetables are soft add the rest of the ingredients except for the cheese. Cover and simmer for 1 hour
3. Serve warm, top with cheese (optional)
4. If you want a chunky dip pour into food processor and pulse, but don't smooth it out
5. Enjoy and scoop chili with celery, carrots, broccoli and

cauliflower florets, freshly cut zucchini or yellow squash sticks

Barely Barley Salad - vegetarian

½ cup pearl barley
½ cup plain low-fat yogurt
1 tbsp fresh lemon juice
2 stalks celery, sliced
¼ cup fresh mint, chopped (optional)
2 bunches arugula, thick stems removed (about 6 cups)
kosher salt and black pepper
2 tbsp extra-virgin olive oil
1 tsp Dijon mustard
1 apple, thinly sliced

1. In a medium saucepan, combine the barley, 1½ cups water, and ½ teaspoon salt and bring to a boil. Reduce heat to medium-low, cover, and simmer until the barley is tender and the water is absorbed, 25 to 30 minutes. Drain and spread on a rimmed baking sheet to cool.
2. Meanwhile, in a large bowl, whisk together the yogurt, oil, lemon juice, mustard, ½ teaspoon salt, and ¼ teaspoon pepper. Add the celery, apple, mint, and cooled barley and toss to combine.
3. Divide the arugula among bowls. Top with the barley mixture.

Crispy Chicken with Roasted Carrots and French Style Green Beans

12 ounces skinless, boneless chicken-breast halves
1 egg, slightly beaten
1 tsp prepared mustard
Dash of black pepper
1 tbsp honey
2 cups cornflakes, finely crushed

1. Preheat oven to 450°F. Cut chicken into 3-by- ¾ inch strips. In a shallow dish, combine egg, honey, and mustard. In another dish, stir together cornflake crumbs and pepper.
2. Dip chicken strips into the egg mixture; roll in crumb mixture to coat. Arrange chicken strips on an ungreased baking sheet.
3. Bake about 12 minutes, or until outsides are golden and chicken is no longer pink.

Yield 4 servings, 212 calories; 23g carbohydrate, 23g protein, 3g fat

Cumin Butternut Cous Cous - vegetarian

1 butternut squash (2 pounds)
1 large yellow onion, diced
¼ tsp cayenne
⅛ tsp ground nutmeg
1 cup canned diced tomatoes
1 32oz container vegetable broth
¼ cup (1 oz) almonds, chopped
2 tbsp chopped fresh flat-leaf parsley leaves
2 tbsp olive oil
2 cloves garlic, finely chopped
⅛ tsp ground cinnamon
1 tsp ground cumin
⅓ cup dark or golden raisins
1 15.5oz can chickpeas, drained
1½ cups couscous
2 tsp kosher salt

1. Halve and peel the squash. Remove the seeds and cut the squash into 1-inch chunks. Heat the oil in a Dutch oven over medium heat. Add the onion and cook for 5 minutes. Add the garlic, cayenne, cinnamon, nutmeg, and ½ teaspoon of the cumin and cook for 1 minute. Stir in the squash, tomatoes, raisins, broth, chickpeas, and 1½ teaspoons of the salt. Bring to a boil. Reduce heat, cover, and simmer for 10 minutes. Uncover and cook until the squash is tender, 15 to 20 minutes.
2. Meanwhile, in a medium saucepan, bring 1½ cups water and the remaining cumin and salt to a boil. Stir in the couscous. Cover, remove from heat, and let stand for 5 to 10 minutes. Fluff with a fork.
3. Divide the couscous among individual bowls and ladle the squash over the top. Sprinkle with the parsley and almonds.

Yield 6-8

Dijon Cheddar Melt with Fruit Salad - low carb

8 slices (½ lb) lean smoked ham, low sodium and nitrate free
4 slices (3oz) reduced-fat aged or sharp cheddar cheese
2 tbsp Dijon mustard
pinch of cayenne (optional)
1 medium tomato sliced

- Line baking tray with foil. Place ham slices on foil and ½ slice of cheese on top, spread the mustard on top and a sprinkle of cayenne, feel free to roll up or leave flat; if you roll up add the tomato prior to rolling, else top with tomato after you've removed from the toaster oven broiler; broil for 4 minutes or until the cheese melts

- Eat hot or cold

Yield 2 servings

Flanking Steak Salad - high protein

¾ pound flank steak
1 head romaine, chopped
1 15.5oz can white beans, rinsed
kosher salt and black pepper
¼ cup chopped parsley
½ cup chopped roasted peppers
¼ small head red cabbage, chopped (about 2 cups)
¼ cup Italian or Vinaigrette dressing

1. Heat broiler. Season steak with ½ teaspoon salt and ¼ teaspoon pepper and place on a broiler proof rimmed baking sheet.
2. Broil the steak, 4 to 5 minutes per side for medium-rare. Let rest for 5 minutes, then cut into ½-inch pieces.
3. Meanwhile, in a large bowl, combine the romaine, cabbage, beans, peppers, and parsley. Add the steak and dressing and toss to combine.

Olive Avocado Salad – paleo, vegetarian

5 cups spring mix salad greens
¾ cup Kalamata olives
½ lemon, juiced
1 tsp rosemary, dried
1½ cup frozen peas, thawed
1 avocado, chopped
½ tbsp olive oil
1 tsp sage, dried
½ tsp salt
½ cup fresh cilantro, torn or loosely chopped

1. Place the mixed greens in a large salad bowl. Top the greens with the olives, avocado, peas and cilantro
2. Drizzle the greens with lemon juice and olive oil
3. Sprinkle with rosemary, sage and salt
4. Toss to combine all ingredients and serve

Yield 6

Cravin'Fit Addition: For more protein, add tofu, turkey breast, roast beef

Crabwich

2 6oz cans of crabmeat or 1 ½ cup of cooked crabmeat
1 cup shredded reduced-fat Swiss or Havarti cheese
¼ cup bell pepper, red or yellow, finally chopped
⅓ cup mashed avocado, or low/non-fat mayonnaise
⅓ cup yellow onion, finely chopped
1½ tsp Dijon mustard
Whole grain/wheat English muffin
½ cup celery, finely chopped
¼ tsp dill, dried

1. Mix crabmeat, celery, onion and bell peppers in a bowl
2. Mixed avocado, mustard and dill in separate small bowl
3. Add the avocado mixture to the crab mixture, combine through
4. Use broiler or toaster oven, top one half of muffin with ¼ of mixture and place in oven until heated through, 2 minutes
5. Top with 2 tbsp of cheese, return to heat until cheese melts
6. Enjoy with baby carrots
7. Refrigerate the remainder, stays fresh for 4 days

Yield 4 servings, 275 calories; 31g carbohydrates, 24g protein, 5g fiber

Giana Grilled Scallops w/Lemon Pepper Zucchini Noodles - low-carb

¾ pound large scallops
2 tsp olive oil
¾ cup Parmesan, freshly grated
¼ cup white wine
4 cups spinach
Salt & freshly ground pepper

1. Preheat oven to 350°F. Place the scallops in a small baking dish, arrange in a single layer. Add the wine, toss and coat the scallops. Bake for 15 minutes
2. Heat oil in a medium nonstick skillet over medium-high heat. Add the spinach and sauté for 2-3 minutes or until wilted. Divide between 2 plates or meal prep containers.
3. Remove scallops from the oven, turn on broiler. When broiler is hot, sprinkle parmesan cheese over the scallops and place under the broiler for 1 minute or until golden, watch carefully as not to burn
4. Season with salt and pepper and serve over spinach

Lemon Pepper Zucchini

½ lb Zucchini Noodles or slices
2 tsp lemon juice, freshly squeeze
2 tsp Olive Oil
¼ tsp black pepper, freshly ground

- In the skillet used for spinach, heat the oil over medium-high heat. Add zucchini and sauté for 5 minutes. Toss with lemon juice and pepper, serve with scallops

Yield 2

Coconut Chicken – high protein

1 cup brown rice, cooked
3oz grilled chicken
2 tbsp unsweetened coconut flakes
¼ cup carrot, chopped or shredded
¼ cup bell pepper (yellow or red), chopped

1. Combine rice and coconut flakes, stir to mix
2. Top with chicken, peppers and carrots
3. Drizzle with Peanut sauce

Mushroom Italia bowl - gluten-free, vegetarian

1 cup cooked quinoa (222 calories)
¼ cup tomato sauce (15 calories)
1 cup cooked mushrooms (28 calories)
½ cup boiled carrots (27 calories)

- Add quinoa to a cute bowl, top with tomato sauce, carrots and mushrooms

Yield 1 serving, 292 calories

Cravin'Fit Addition: add ¼ cup of diced chicken breast for more protein, it only add 55

Red Light Lentil Soup – high fiber, high protein

3 tbsp olive oil
½ cup red onion
½ cup green pepper, chopped
½ cup red pepper, chopped
3 jalapeños
6 garlic cloves
3 medium tomatoes, diced
4 celery stalks
4 cups of water
1 sprig of marjoram
2 cups dried red lentils, soaked overnight and rinsed
4 cups reduced/low sodium chicken stock

1. In a 4qt pan heat oil, onion, peppers, jalapenos, and garlic
2. Sauté until onions are translucent
3. Add lentils, tomatoes, celery, chicken stock and water; bring to a boil for 2 minutes.
4. Cover and simmer for 20minutes or until lentils are slightly crunchy
5. Pour soup into a blender and blend on low, stop when you get the perfect ratio of chunkiness
6. Serve with pita bread or homemade pita chips

Yield 4-6, serving size 1 cup 388 calories; carbohydrates 55g, protein 23g, fat 10g, fiber 11g, sodium 467mg, sugars 5g

Greek Heart Bowl - gluten-free, vegetarian

1 cup cooked quinoa (222 calories)
12 artichoke hearts (90 calories)
½ cup cucumber slices (8 calories)
1 tbsp balsamic vinegar (10 calories)

- Layer ingredients in a bowl starting with quinoa, artichokes, cucumbers and dress with Balsamic or Greek Vinaigrette

Yield 1 serving, 330 calories

Sun-Dried Turkey Pita

6 slices of turkey breast meat, Low sodium and nitrate free
2 tbsp plain Greek Yogurt, or Mayonnaise, or mashed avocado
2 tbsp sun-dried tomatoes, drained and diced
½ cup reduced-fat mozzarella cheese
3 tbsp capers, drained
Handful of spinach sundried

Whole wheat or whole grain pita

1. Combine sun-dried tomatoes, Greek yogurt and capers together in a small bowl
2. Cut pita in half, stuff the pita with turkey breast, the sun-dried tomato mixture, spinach and cheese use a toaster oven to broil until cheese is bubbly, serve hot
3. Enjoy with a honeycrisp apple

Yield 2

White Bean and Rice Salad - vegetarian

1 cup brown rice, cooked
¼ cup cherry tomatoes
1 tbsp olive oil
1 tsp garlic, minced
¼ cup white beans
1 tbsp chopped dill
1½ lemon juice

- Toss together rice and white beans and cherry tomatoes with dill and olive oil and lemon juice and minced garlic

Portobello Arugula Salad - gluten-free, vegetarian, vegan

4 cups arugula, rinsed and dried
1 cup balsamic vinegar
3 large Portobello mushrooms
1 tablespoon turbinado sugar
1 tsp gluten-free low sodium soy sauce or Bragg's Liquid Aminos

1. Put arugula in a big salad bowl
2. Clean mushrooms and remove stems, grill for 10minutes or use a grill pan turn once, place mushroom caps atop arugula
3. Heat the vinegar, sugar, and soy sauce in a small saucepan to a boil. Reduce heat to low and simmer for 15-20 minutes, or until ingredients thicken. Remove from heat and let cool.
4. Once balsamic glaze has cooled a bit, pour evenly over mushrooms and arugula. Enjoy immediately or wait for the glaze to cool a few more minutes

Yield 6 servings

Salmon Poppy Bowl - gluten-free, high protein

¾ cup cooked quinoa (167 calories)
4 oz smoked/grilled/steamed salmon (133 calories)
¼ cup nonfat Greek yogurt (33 calories)
2 tsp poppy seeds (29 calories)

- Combine layer salmon over the quinoa in a bowl, top with yogurt and poppy seeds

Yield 1 serving; 362 calories

West Indian Chicken and Rice - diabetic friendly, high protein

1 (8oz) can pineapple tidbits in their own juice, drained
½ cup fat-free, low-sodium chicken broth
2 boneless skinless chicken breast halves (4oz each)
2 tsp low sodium soy sauce or Bragg's Liquid Aminos
½ cup uncooked instant brown rice
2 medium green onions, thinly sliced
2 tbsp red bell peppers, diced
1 tsp jerk seasoning, salt-free

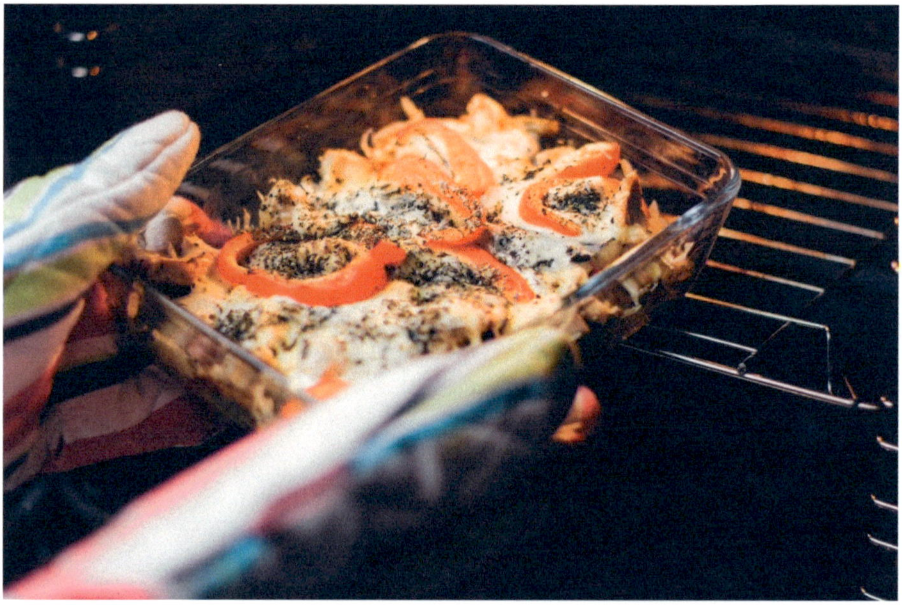

1. Preheat oven to 375°F
2. In an 8-ince square baking pan, stir together the pineapple, broth, rice, green onions and bell pepper

3. Sprinkle seasoning over both sides of chicken, place the chicken atop the pineapple mixture. Pour the soy sauce over the chicken
4. Bake, covered for 40-45minutes, or until the chicken is no longer pink in the center and the rice is tender.

Yield 2, Serving size 3oz chicken breast and 1 cup of fruit and rice, Calories; 365, 30g protein 4g fat, 4g fiber, 13g sugar, sodium 295mg

Mexi-Cali bowl - gluten-free, vegetarian

¾ cup cooked quinoa (167 calories)
⅓ cup black beans (76 calories)
½ avocado (114 calories)
2 tbsp pico de gallo (10 calories)

- Combine ingredients in a bowl and enjoy with a small peach

Yield 1 serving, 367 calories

Gumbo over Wild Rice or Quinoa - gluten-free

2 tbsp brown rice flour (or whole wheat flour if you aren't following a gluten free diet)
2 tbsp butter or olive oil
4 cloves garlic, diced
2 carrots, diced
1 quart chicken broth, gluten-free
2 cups okra, diced
1 large green bell pepper, diced
1 medium onion, diced
2 stalks celery, diced
2 tbsp Cajun seasoning, gluten-free
1½ cups fresh tomatoes, diced
4 chicken Andouille sausage, sliced, gluten-free

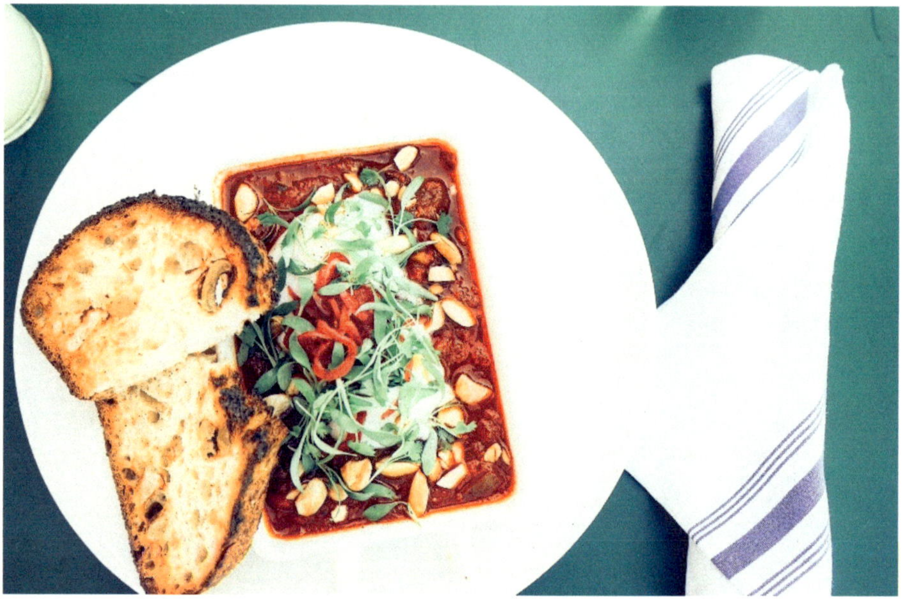

1. In a nonstick skillet, melt the butter. Add the flour and stir until the flour is golden brown. Add the pepper, garlic, onion, carrots and celery. Sauté 3-5 minutes
2. Add the mixture to a 4 quart slow cooker. Add the broth, seasoning, sausage and tomatoes, cook on low for 8-10 hours
3. Add okra for the last hour of cooking. Stir prior to serving.

Yield 8

21 Cravin'Fit SNACKS

KEY:

DF – diabetic friendly	**GF** – gluten-free
LC – low carb	**HP** – high protein
P – paleo	**VE** – vegan
VG – vegetarian	

Bruschetta Caps - gluten free, vegetarian

6 large Portobello mushrooms caps, wiped clean, stems removed
6 plum/roma tomatoes, seeded and chopped

2 tbsp Extra Virgin Olive Oil	½ red onion, chopped finely
4 cloves garlic, minced	2 tbsp balsamic vinegar
3 tbsp fresh basil, torn	8oz fresh mozzarella, thinly sliced
½ tsp sea salt	½ tsp pepper
1 tbsp Parmesan cheese, grated	Oil Mister filled with Olive Oil

1. Preheat oven to 425°F, spray a baking sheet with cooking spray
2. In a large bowl, combine tomatoes, olive oil, onion, garlic, vinegar, basil and parmesan cheese. Add salt and pepper and mix well
3. Slice each mushroom cap in half; you should have 2 half circles, place on baking sheet, mist with olive oil or lightly drizzle with olive oil. Bake for 5 minutes and remove from oven
4. Spoon bruschetta on each mushroom half. Top with mozzarella and bake for 2-3 minutes until cheese is melted

Creole Plaintain Chips - vegan, vegetarian

¼ cup of Creole season (or make your own; paprika + chili powder + red pepper flakes and cayenne)
4 large green plantains (2 lbs)
Brown paper bag
Coconut oil for frying

1. Peel the plantains and slice then thin slice the fruit or use a mandolin or any other fancy kitchen slicing device
2. Measure 1 tbsp of Creole seasoning put it the paper bag
3. Warm a large pan with coconut oil over medium-high heat
4. Place slices of plantain in the oil in a single layer, fry only 1 plantain at a time. Cook evenly on both sides for about a minute
5. Remove the slices with a round skimmer when they are golden and place directly into the brown plastic bag
6. Shake to evenly coat the plantain chips
7. Place seasoned chips on a paper towel lined plate.

8. Repeat until all of the plantains are cooked.

Yield 4

Cranberry Pecan Balls - vegan

1 cup pitted Medjool dates
½ cup raw pecans
⅛ tsp ground ginger
1 cup unsweetened dried cranberries
1 cup raw almonds
¼ tsp ground cinnamon
⅛ fine sea salt

1. In a small glass bowl place dates and enough boiled water to cover them. Seal the top, aluminum foil or a larger plate will do. Let them soak for 5 minutes. Drain
2. Place almonds, pecans, cinnamon, ginger and salt in a food processor. Pulse the ingredients until they are finely ground.
3. Add the dates and process until it is thoroughly blended and visibly sticky
4. Scoop ingredients into a larger bowl, add the cranberries and hand mix
5. Time to clean your hands and Get your roll on, but leave your hands a little wet
6. Roll the Balls into about 1" remember you have to get 12 out of them, so no gigantic balls
7. If your hands start to stick together, wet them again and keep rolling
8. Feel free to eat right away, but they can be kept for no longer than 1 month in an airtight container

Yield 12, 1 ball is a serving

Healthy Spinach Artichoke Dip - vegetarian

1 (13.75oz) can of artichoke hearts packed in water, drained and chopped
10 oz frozen spinach, thawed and squeezed
½ cup mashed avocado, get as many chunks out as possible
¼ cup shallots, chopped
½ cup Greek yogurt, plain
4 oz shredded part skim-mozzarella
Tabasco sauce
1 garlic clove chopped
2/3 cup grated Parmesan cheese
Salt & Pepper to taste
Red pepper flakes

1. In a large bowl blend the artichoke hearts and spinach. Add a few drops of Tabasco sauce (optional) set aside

2. Sauté the shallots in olive oil until translucent. Then add chopped garlic and sauté for one more minute. Remove from heat
3. Add sautéed veggies to spinach artichoke mixture
4. Add avocado, Greek yogurt, shredded mozzarella cheese and Paramesan cheese to spinach artichoke mixture and blend well
5. Season with salt and pepper and red pepper flakes
6. Spread into an oiled casserole dish and sprinkle leftover cheese on top
7. Bake at 350°F until lightly brown and bubbly, serve warm with homemade pita chips or pita bread (whole grain) and carrots and broccoli

Nut Butter Multigrain Crackers - vegetarian

1 small banana
1 tbsp nut butter of your choice to spread on crackers
6-10 Multigrain or whole wheat crackers

Bump on a Banana Log - vegan

1 banana
Sprinkle of cinnamon
1 tbsp almond butter
1 tbsp salted pistachios, chopped

1. Peel the banana and smear one side with the almond butter.
2. Sprinkle with cinnamon and chopped nuts.
3. Slice and enjoy!

Yield 2 servings, 114 calories; 15g carbohydrates , protein 2.7g, 5.6g fat, fiber 2.1g, sugars 7.4g 11g sodium,

No Slack PB Flax Squares - gluten free

1 cup dry old-fashioned gluten-free oats
½ cup natural peanut butter, gluten free
½ cup dark chocolate chips
⅓ cup honey
½ cup ground flaxseed
1 tsp vanilla extract

1. Stir all ingredients together in a medium-sized bowl until thoroughly mixed

2. Spread mixture in a 9x9" pan and refrigerate for an hour
3. Cut into small squares. Keeps for 1 week stored in an airtight container in the refrigerator
4. *Optional Additions:* your favorite ingredients like dried cranberries, goji berries, raisins, nuts, coconut flakes

Pump Smoothie

1 cup organic vanilla soymilk/almond milk (or preferred milk substitute)
½ cup Pure Canned Pumpkin (or fresh)
½ cup low-fat/no-fat vanilla yogurt
½ cup unsweetened applesauce
½ scoop (15g) vanilla whey protein
½ tbsp ground cinnamon
1 cup of ice

- Place all ingredients in blender and blend until smooth

Honey, Pass The Peas - vegan

15oz can organic chickpeas (aka garbanzo beans)
½ tbsp olive oil
1 tbsp honey
½ tsp cinnamon
⅛ tsp nutmeg
⅛ tsp sea salt

1. Preheat oven to 375°F. Line baking sheet with parchment paper
2. Drain and rinse the chickpeas. Place them on a plate lined with paper towels to dry
3. Spread on lined baking sheet, single layer. Bake for 45mins or until crispy. Check the peas, if they are still soft bake a little longer
4. When the chickpeas are done quickly mix the remaining ingredients in a medium sized bowl, and toss the chickpeas in the mixture, making sure to get a good coating
5. Put the honey coated pea mixture back in the oven for 10 minutes
6. Keep in an airtight container after cooling or get your plastic bags out for meal prep

Yield 4 servings

Kale Chips - gluten-free, paleo, vegetarian

1 lb (2 large bunches) Kale, washed stemmed, and dried thoroughly
2 tbsp coconut oil
Favorite seasoning – Chipotle, Cajun, Lemon-Pepper

1. Preheat oven to 350°F
2. Make sure the kale leaves are dry, drier than a dessert in Arizona dry! Feel free to use paper towels to pat dry them
3. Toss the dried leaves with oil, get hands-on to make sure the oil is distributed evenly. Arrange the leaves in a single layer, with space between the leaves, on parchment lined baking sheets; you may need more than one. Sprinkle season on now or when they come out, exercise your personal preference.
4. Bake each tray for 12 minutes on the middle rack until crispy, not burnt.

Yield 3 cups

Mango-Chia Pudding – gluten-free, vegetarian

2 mangoes peeled and pitted
3 tbsp chia seeds
½ cup light/low-cal coconut milk
1 tbsp agave

1. Blend mangoes, milk and agave until smooth
2. Add 3 tbsp chia seeds, mix until evenly distributed 1-3 seconds
3. Pour into 2 bowls or ramekin sized dishes
4. Refrigerate for 30mins or overnight

Refresh Juice – gluten-free, vegetarian

1 medium cucumber, chopped
¾ cup kale, torn or chopped
½ lemon, remove seeds
½ apple, medium to large, chopped
½ pear, medium, chopped
½ cup of water, or more for desired consistency

- Blend all ingredients until smooth

Yield: 1 serving, 173 calories, 4g of protein, 8g of fiber, 25g of sugar

Salt & Vinegar Chicks - gluten-free, vegan, vegetarian

2 cups canned chickpeas
1 tsp Coarse sea salt
3-4 cups white vinegar, or regular
2 tsp extra virgin olive oil

1. Line a baking sheet with tin foil or parchment paper.
2. Take chickpeas and vinegar and place in a medium sized pot. Add a dash of sea salt. Bring to a boil and then remove from heat. Let sit in pot for 30 minutes.
3. Preheat oven to 400°F
4. Carefully drain chickpeas.
5. Place on lined baking sheet and drizzle with olive oil and sea salt. Massage with fingers until fully coated. Roast for 30-40 minutes, flipping once half way through. Keep an eye on them after 25 minutes of cooking so they don't burn.

What's Up Doc? Energy Balls - vegetarian

⅓ cup coconut flakes, sweetened or unsweetened
⅔ cup grated carrot (1 large carrot)
½ tsp ground cinnamon
heaping ¼ cup dried pineapple
heaping ¼ cup toasted pecans, chopped
½ cup coconut flakes for rolling (optional)
2 tbsp flaxseed meal
⅓ cup old-fashioned oats
¼ tsp ground ginger
½ tsp vanilla extract
4 large dates

1. In the bowl of your food processor (or blender), add grated carrot, coconut flakes, flaxseed meal, oats, cinnamon, and ginger. Pulse to combine.
2. Add dates, dried pineapple, pecans, and vanilla extract. Pulse until the mixture comes together. You'll know the mixture is ready when it forms a slight dough ball in the bowl of your food processor.
3. Shape the mixture in to tablespoon-size balls. Roll the balls in coconut flakes. Store in an airtight container, separating the layers with parchment or wax paper. Refrigerate for at least an hour before serving.

Yield: 10 energy balls

Tortilla Pizza – low-carb

1 low-carb tortilla, (brown rice, whole wheat, or whole grain)
1½ tbsp no-sugar added pizza sauce (Ragu)
½ cup shredded mozzarella cheese
Any additional toppings, turkey pepperoni, broccoli, mushrooms

1. Place tortilla on the tray of a toaster oven. Spread pizza sauce over it, then top with cheese
2. Bake in toaster oven at 450°F until the cheese is bubbly and starting to brown, cut into wedges and enjoy

Dip Me at the Greek – vegetarian

1 6oz container strained Greek yogurt
1-2 cucumbers, cut into ½" wedges
¼ bunch flat-leaf Italian parsley, chopped
½ bunch chives, thinly sliced
Lemon juice to taste
Salt to taste
1 clove garlic

1. Chop garlic, then add a generous pinch of coarse salt. Mash the garlic and salt mixture with the flat side of your knife.
2. Stir garlic paste, chives, parsley, and lemon juice into Greek yogurt until well combined. Salt to taste.
3. Serve with cucumber wedges or vegetables of your choice.

Caliente Black Bean Hummus – vegetarian

1 small jalapeño pepper, chopped (or ½ tsp cayenne pepper)
15 oz black beans, rinsed and drained
1 tbsp tahini
2 tbsp olive oil
Salt and pepper to taste
Juice from 1 lemon
1 clove garlic

1. Add the garlic and jalapeño to a food processor or blender and puree. Add in the remaining ingredients and mix until smooth.
2. Enjoy immediately or store in an airtight glass container in the fridge for up to a week.

Parmesan Zucchini Sticks – gluten-free, low-carb, vegetarian

1 cup zucchini, sliced into 2-3" sticks
Oil Mister (optional) with Olive Oil
Salt and pepper to taste
Non stick cooking spray
1 tbsp Shaved Parmesan

1. Preheat oven on broil, line baking sheet with aluminum foil and spray with cooking spray
2. Placed sliced zucchini sticks on aluminum foil and spray lightly, or lightly drizzle olive oil over sticks
3. Sprinkle parmesan cheese on top of sticks, season with salt and pepper
4. Broil for a few minutes until cheese melts and turns light brown, 2 minutes

Sweet Potato Fries – gluten-free, paleo, vegetarian

6 sweet potatoes peeled and cut into wedges, about 1 inch
4 tsp olive oil
Cinnamon, Cumin and Cayenne
Sea salt to taste

1. Preheat oven to 350°F. Line a baking sheet with aluminum foil
2. In a large bowl mix wedges with oil and seasoning
3. Spread wedges on baking sheet in a single layer bake for 30-45, they should be crispy on the outside and give when you press them

Thai Cabbage Wontons – high protein

1 pound ground chicken
1 cup cabbage chopped
¼ cup sliced scallions
Juice from 1 lime
2 tbsp vegetable oil for brushing
1 tbsp fish sauce, lite soy sauce, or Bragg Liquid Aminos
½ medium red onion, chopped
½ cup chopped cilantro
Red pepper flakes
48 wonton wrappers

1. Preheat oven to 400°F. With a brush, lightly oil a baking sheet.
2. Heat medium-sized skillet, and add two tablespoons of

water. Add ground chicken and cook until almost done.

3. Add chopped onion and lettuce, and cook until onion is translucent and lettuce is slightly wilted.
4. Add fish sauce, cilantro, scallions, and pepper flakes; stir and cook until scallions and cilantro are slightly wilted. Remove from heat and add lime juice, mixing thoroughly. Adjust seasoning if necessary.
5. Drain mixture in colander, and set aside to cool.
6. To make the wontons, place wonton wrapper in front of you in a diamond shape, and spoon one teaspoon of the cooled filling in the center. Wet the edges of the wonton wrapper with water, and fold the end closest to you over the filling to make a triangle; press ends together. Take the left and right ends of the triangle, and wet with water; fold them together over the center of the wonton, and press to seal.
7. Place wontons on baking sheet; once filled, lightly brush the wontons with oil.
8. Bake wontons for 10 minutes; you may want to put them under the broiler for a couple minutes to brown even more.
9. Serve with hot sauce, soy sauce, or a fish-sauce-based dipping sauce like this

Calories per wonton: 43 calories per

Go Goji Choco bowl – gluten-free

¼ cup cooked quinoa (56 calories)
2 tbsp coconut flakes (50 calories)
1½ tbsp goji berries (52 calories)
1 tbsp dark chocolate chips (melted) (70 calories)

- Combine ingredients in a bowl and enjoy, feel free to add a dollop of Greek yogurt

Yield 1 serving; 228 calories

21 Cravin'Fit DINNERS

KEY:

DF – diabetic friendly
LC – low carb
P – paleo
VG – vegetarian
GF – gluten-free
HP – high protein
VE – vegan

Balsamic Pear Bowl - low fat, vegetarian

1 cup brown rice, cooked
½ tsp sage leaf, chopped
2 tsp balsamic glaze
½ pear, chopped
2 tbsp crumbled gorgonzola

- Combine rice pear, sage and gorgonzola in a bowl, drizzle with balsamic glaze

Cravin'Fit Additions: For more protein add in ½-⅓ cup of chickpeas

Beet the Feta Salad - diabetic friendly, low carb, vegetarian

2 medium beets, peeled and chopped
1½ oz baby arugula; approx 1½ cups
¼ tsp Dijon Mustard
2 tsp olive oil
½ tsp white wine vinegar

- In a large bowl, whisk olive oil, vinegar, and mustard. Add the arugula, use a tong to twirl the leaves throughout dressing. Add beets, sprinkle with feta, toss for combine.

Yield 2 servings, 105 calories; 8g carbohydrate, 7g protein, 5g fat, 5g sugars

Cravin'Fit Additions: Goes great with 3-6oz of grilled beef tenderloin or spicy baby back ribs

Chicken Tortilla Soup – gluten-free

2 cups cubed cooked boneless chicken breast
14oz canned fire-roasted diced tomatoes
3 cups chicken broth, gluten free
2 habañero peppers, seeded and diced
4oz canned diced green chilies, drained
1 cup fresh corn kernels
2 cloves garlic, minced
25oz canned crush tomatoes
1 tsp chili powder, gluten free
⅛ tsp salt
1 medium onion, diced
1 tsp cumin
1 tsp smoked paprika

1. Place cumin, chili powder, paprika, salt, tomatoes, broth, garlic, onion, chilies and peppers in a 4qt slow cooker. Cover and cook on low for 6 hours
2. Add corn and cooked chicken. Cover and cook for an

additional 45-60minutes

Tortilla strips

Slice 4 gluten-free corn tortillas in half, then into ¼ inch strips. Heat ½ tsp canola oil in a shallow skillet. Add tortilla strips and cook, turning once, until crisps and golden, when done place on paper towel lined plate and blot to remove excess oil, Top soup with strips

Yield 8

Curried Lamb with Coconut Piña Rice - gluten-free, paleo, low carb

1 lb lamb, lean cut, cut into chunks
1 tsp curry powder, gluten-free
4 cloves garlic, minced
2 tsp hot sauce,
½ cup peanut oil
2 tbsp lemon juice
½ tsp ground coriander

1. Mix peanut oil, curry, lemon juice, garlic, coriander and hot sauce together in a bowl
2. Add lamb, toss to coat. Cover and refrigerate for 2 hours
3. Pour lamb and marinade into a medium non-stick skillet, cook on medium-high heat for 10 minutes or until desired doneness, stirring occasionally

Yield 4 servings

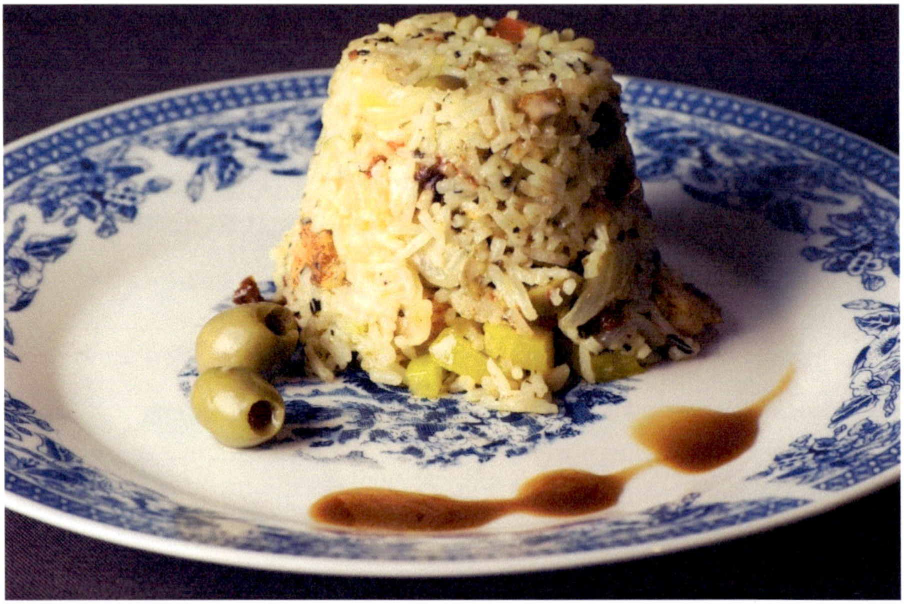

Coconut Piña rice **(gluten-free, low carb, paleo, vegetarian)**

1 medium cauliflower head, cut into pieces to fit your food processor
1 cup fresh pineapple diced ¼" cubes
2 tbsp coconut oil, or favorite oil
½ cup full-fat coconut milk
1 small yellow onion, minced
1 scallion, thinly sliced
Freshly ground pepper

1. Process cut cauliflower in a food processor, pulse and process until it resembles rice
2. Melt coconut oil on medium-high heat in a large skillet, sauté onion for 5 minutes or until translucent and season with a pinch of salt
3. Add the cauliflower and coconut milk to the skillet and stir evenly to mix thoroughly. Season with salt to taste (optional) Cover and cook for 5-10 more minutes until the mixture has absorbed the coconut milk, the rice should be tender and fluffy
4. Remove the rice from the stove and put in a large bowl. Add the pineapple and scallions, mix through. Sprinkle with pepper and kosher salt

Yield 6 servings

Lentil Kale salad - gluten-free, vegetarian

1 tbsp Extra Virgin olive oil
¼ cup onion, chopped
½ cup tomatoes, sliced
½ tsp kosher salt
2 tbsp lemon juice, fresh
3 cloves garlic, chopped
2 cups Kale, stems removed
1-2 tbsp fresh basil
8oz lentils, cooked and soaked
2 tbsp shaved Asiago cheese

1. Heat oil in a large skillet over medium-high heat. Add garlic and onion and sauté for 2 minutes
2. Add kale and tomatoes and sauté for 2-3 minutes more until kale is softened but still crisp. Add basil and salt and stir until blended
3. In a large bowl combine the kale mixture with the cooked lentils, still well
4. Stir in lemon juice and cheese. Serve hot or cold

Yield 6

Ginger Halibut with Lemon Tahini Cauliflower - high protein, low carb

½ lb Halibut
¼ tsp ginger
1 garlic clove, chopped
½ tsp olive oil

1. Turn the broiler on the oven, line a baking sheet or broiler pan with aluminum foil, stick it in the oven alone for 5 minutes
2. Take it out place fish in the pan, dress with ginger, garlic and olive oil then return to the oven. broil for 8-10 minutes

Lemon Tahini dressing

¼ cup tahini
½ lemon juiced
¼ cup white miso
Hot water

1. Whisk ingredients together adding water to reach perfect consistency
2. Pour over steamed cauliflower

Chicken Piccata – high protein

2 boneless chicken breast
¼ cup rice flour, or whole wheat flour
1 tsp olive oil
1 tbsp capers

¼ cup chopped flat-leaf parsley
1 tbsp lemon juice, freshly squeezed
¾ cup dry white wine
¼ tsp sea salt
¼ tsp pepper

1. Flatten chicken breast with a mallet to about ¼ inch thickness
2. Combine flour, salt and pepper
3. Coat chicken in flour mixture
4. Heat olive oil in skillet over medium-high heat.
5. Add chicken, cook 3minutes on each side until browned
6. Add half of the wine, the juice and the capers to the pan, scraping the pan to loosen any brown bits
7. Cook 2 minutes
8. Remove chicken from the pan, but keep warm
9. Stir in rest of wine and cook until it is reduced by half, Stir in fresh chopped parsley
10. Serve with wild rice and asparagus

Yield 2, Serving is 1 Chicken Breast, calories 298, 29g of protein

Crab and Avocado Salad - gluten-free, low-carb

Dressing

2 tbsp lime juice, fresh
1 tsp cilantro, chopped
½ tsp Old Bay Season
2 tbsp lemon juice, fresh
4 tbsp pineapple juice
1 tbsp olive oil

Salad

12 oz lump crabmeat (blue, Dungeness or king)
¼ head dark green lettuce, shredded
½ avocado, peeled and diced
¼ cup red pepper, diced
1 medium tomato

1. Combine the dressing ingredients in a small bowl
2. Mix the pepper, avocado and tomatoes in a medium mixing bowl until well combined. Fold in crabmeat, be gentle you don't want it to separate more than natural
3. Put a cup of shredded lettuce in large bowl and toss with ¼ cup dressing then transfer to serving bowls
4. Divide crabmeat into four then place atop lettuce
5. Pour 1 tbsp dressing on each serving, there will be extra

dressing left over, use as needed

Yield 4 servings, Serving Size ¼ salad, calories 180; 8g carbohydrates, 8.5g fat, 19g protein, 4g sugars

Taco Boats - high protein

1lb ground 93-95% lean turkey or beef
1 tsp Garlic
1 tsp Chili powder
1 tsp Mexican season
1 tsp Cumin
4 Romaine lettuce leaves

fixings

½ Avocado, chopped
½ cup low-fat Mexican cheese
Banana peppers
1 plum tomato, chopped
Salsa or picante sauce

1. Brown meat over medium-high heat, stirring often to crumble meat, drain when done
2. Return to pan add seasons and mix thoroughly,
3. Put ⅓ cup of meat in each romaine leaf, then top with toppings
4. Serve with Roasted Corn and lemon cilantro brown rice
5. ** **

Cravin'Fit Swap: Vegetarians swap black beans for meat

Soy Chicken with Kale – gluten-free, low-carb

4 tbsp low-sodium gluten-free soy sauce, or Bragg's Liquid Aminos
2 boneless, skinless chicken breasts, cut into 1" cut cubes
1 tbsp toasted sesame oil
½ tsp gingerroot, freshly grated
1 tbsp Extra Virgin Olive Oil
1 tbsp honey
2 cloves garlic, crushed
2 cups Kale

1. In a small bowl, whisk together the soy sauce, sesame oil, honey, gingerroot and garlic
2. Place chicken in zip-top plastic bag and pour half of the mixture into the bag. Seal bag tight. Shake the bag so the chicken is covered. Marinate for an hour or overnight.
3. Remove chicken from marinade. Heat olive oil in a skillet over medium-high heat. Sauté the chicken for 5-8minutes, until

fully cooked and no longer pink

4. Add the kale and cook until it is till bright green but only a little soft, approx 2 minutes. Add remaining soy mixture and mix well.

Yield 2

Tandoori Shrimp Fry – high protein, paleo, low carb

1½ lb shrimp, wild-caught, peeled and deveined
1 tbsp olive oil
1 red bell pepper, diced
½ tsp salt
1 tbsp Tandoori spice
1 tbsp Coconut aminos
1 small yellow onion, diced
1 tsp garlic powder
½ tsp black pepper
½ tsp red pepper flakes
Shredded Cabbage

1. In a large skillet melt oil over medium-heat
2. Add onion and bell pepper, sauté until onions are translucent
3. Add shrimp to the skillet until the shrimp is no longer pink or translucent
4. Season with garlic powder, salt, pepper and tandoori spice, red pepper flakes, coconut aminos, stir until the shrimp are completely seasoned
5. Serve over shredded cabbage, purple cabbage is prettier on a plate

Yield 4 servings

Tomato Basil Sea Bass with Steamed Asparagus – gluten-free

4 cups canned tomato puree no added salt
4 4-oz sea bass filets
4 cups chopped tomatoes
4 tbsp fresh basil, minced
4 tsp shallots, minced *approx 4
1 tsp salt
1 tsp pepper
4 tsp olive oil

1. Rub each filet with olive oil, sprinkle each with ¼ tsp of salt and pepper
2. In a large bowl mix together chopped tomatoes, puree, and 3 tbsp of basil and shallots
3. Place fish in a large skillet or baking dish. Pour the sauce of the fish. Bake at 375° for 5 minutes, or until fish flakes easily

when tested with a fork

4. Sprinkle the remaining tablespoon of basil and shallots over the fish and serve hot.

Yield 4 servings, Serving size: 1 filet with sauce, calories 323; 33g carbohydrate, 33g protein, 8g fat, 8g fiber

Ginger Carrot Soup and Cucumber Salad – gluten-free, vegetarian

6 cups diced carrots
1 cup orange juice, preferably fresh
2 tbsp minced ginger
1 tsp stevia, or substitute
½ tsp white pepper
6 cups vegetable broth, low sodium
3 small onions, diced
1 tsp coconut oil
¼ tsp sea salt
¼ cup chopped cilantro

1. In a large pot, sauté the onion in oil until translucent. Once the onions are soft add the carrots and ginger, sauté for an additional minute
2. Add vegetable broth, cook until carrots are tender
3. Transfer liquid to food processor or blender to puree, then add puree bad to pot, pour in the orange juice and sugar, stir with a spoon
4. Season with salt and pepper, add more water or broth if the consistency is too thick
5. Ladle 1 cup into a bowl and top with cilantro

Yield 6 cups, Serving size 1 cup, 2g fat, 5g protein, 5g fiber

Cucumber Salad

1 large cucumber, sliced
¼ cup feta
Balsamic Vinegar or glaze
¼ cup red onion, thinly sliced,
2 tbsp sunflower seeds

- Combine all ingredients except vinegar in bowl or small serving dish then drizzle with balsamic

Oodles of Noodles – Pork - gluten-free, high protein, low-fat

1 oz uncooked thin rice noodles, available in ethnic section of grocery store
6 fresh snow peas, trimmed and cut into ¼ inch pieces
1 tsp low-sodium soy sauce or Bragg's Liquid Aminos
1½ cups fat-free, low-sodium chicken broth
1 medium green onion, thinly sliced
½ medium carrot, shredded

1 tsp toasted sesame oil
2 cups boiling water

1. Put rice noodles in a medium glass bowl. Pour in boiling water. Cover with plastic wrap. Let stand for 10minutes. Drain in a colander. [* use kitchen scissors to cut and separate noodles]
2. Put snow peas, carrots, and green onion in 2 bowls. Drizzle the soy sauce and sesame oil over the vegetables
3. When the noodles are almost ready, in a small saucepan, bring the broth to a rolling boil
4. Get your tongs out and divide the noodles between the bowls. Pour the boiling broth into the bowls, stir just to combine. Let Stand for 2 minutes, or until the vegetables are tender-crisp
5. Top with 4 oz of sliced or cubed tenderloin from below, or 4 oz of protein, beans, tofu, etc.

Yield 2

Tenderloin

1lb pork tenderloin
Seasoned with onions, garlic, ginger, and Sriracha (hot sauce)
1 tbsp fresh ginger, peeled and finely chopped or grated
¼ cup low-sodium soy sauce or Bragg's Liquid Aminos
½ lime, juiced
¼ cup rice vinegar

1. Combine ginger, soy sauce, lime juice and zest, (2 Tbsp.) oil and grill seasoning in a large sealable plastic bag.
2. Add pork tenderloin to marinade and coat evenly. Let stand 30 minutes to an hour, overnight is even better.
3. 1 lb or .75lb pork tenderloin
4. Preheat oven to 425 degrees.

5. Heat 1 Tbsp. olive oil in a large skillet over medium-high heat.
6. Add to the skillet and cook, turning as needed, for 4 to 5 minutes (about 1 minute per side), until evenly browned.

7. Transfer tenderloin to a greased baking dish, and brush some of the reserved marinade evenly over the tenderloin.
8. Place the dish in the oven to roast for 12 to 15 minutes,
9. Check doneness - if you have a thermometer insert into the thickest part of the tenderloin reads 140 degrees.
10. Remove dish from oven and transfer the tenderloin to a plate and cover loosely with aluminum foil to keep warm.

Pork: 163 calories, protein 29g, total fat 4g | Noodle Bowl: 105 calories, 3g fat

Sadie Jane's Seafood Stew - gluten-free, high protein, low-carb

1 lb of shrimp, 20-40 count (uncooked, peeled, and deveined)
1 lb of haddock fillets (sliced into 1-inch pieces)
1 can of clams (chopped and undrained)
1 can of tomatoes (diced and undrained)
1 can of crabmeat (drained)
3 celery sticks (chopped)
1 can of tomato paste
5 cloves of garlic (minced)
1 tbsp of olive oil
2 tbsp of parsley (minced)
½ tsp of sugar substitute of choice
2 onions (chopped)
1 bottle of clam juice
½ cup of vegetable broth
1 tbsp of red wine vinegar
1 tsp of Italian seasoning
1 bay leaf

1. Combine the tomatoes, onions, celery sticks, clam juice, tomato paste, vegetable broth, garlic, red wine vinegar, olive oil, bay leaf, Italian seasoning, and sugar in a slow cooker and cook on low heat for 5 hours.
2. Add in shrimp, crabmeat, and clams into the slow cooker, cover it, and let it cook for 30 minutes more.
3. Discard the bay leaf, garnish with parsley, and serve.

Olive Turkey Pesto – high protein, low carb, paleo

1 lb ground turkey, 93-95% lean
1 ½ tbsp olive oil
1 cup Kalamata olives
½ yellow onion, diced
1 tsp garlic powder

1. Heat olive oil in a large skillet over medium-heat
2. Add the diced onion and sauté until the onion is soft
3. Add the ground turkey to the skillet, season with salt, pepper and garlic powder, sauté until done, drain and set aside

***Pesto Squash* – (low carb)**

2lb spaghetti squash
1 clove garlic, smashed
½ cup lemon juice
½ cup olive oil (or ¼ cup oil ¼ cup avocado)
2 cups fresh basil, packed
⅓ cup pine nuts
½ tsp salt

1. Preheat oven to 400°F
2. Cut the squash in half lengthwise, discard the seeds
3. Spray a baking sheet with cooking spray, place squash halves cut-side down
4. Bake for 40mins
5. Take a fork and scrape the insides out into a large bowl and toss with pesto below

Pesto

1. Add basil, garlic and pine nuts to a food processor and pulse together. Add lemon juice, olive oil and salt to the process and blend until smooth. Set aside to mix with spaghetti squash.
2. Transfer pesto squash to a serving dish stir in ground turkey and top with olives

Yield 8 servings, 6g of carbohydrates (squash noodles)

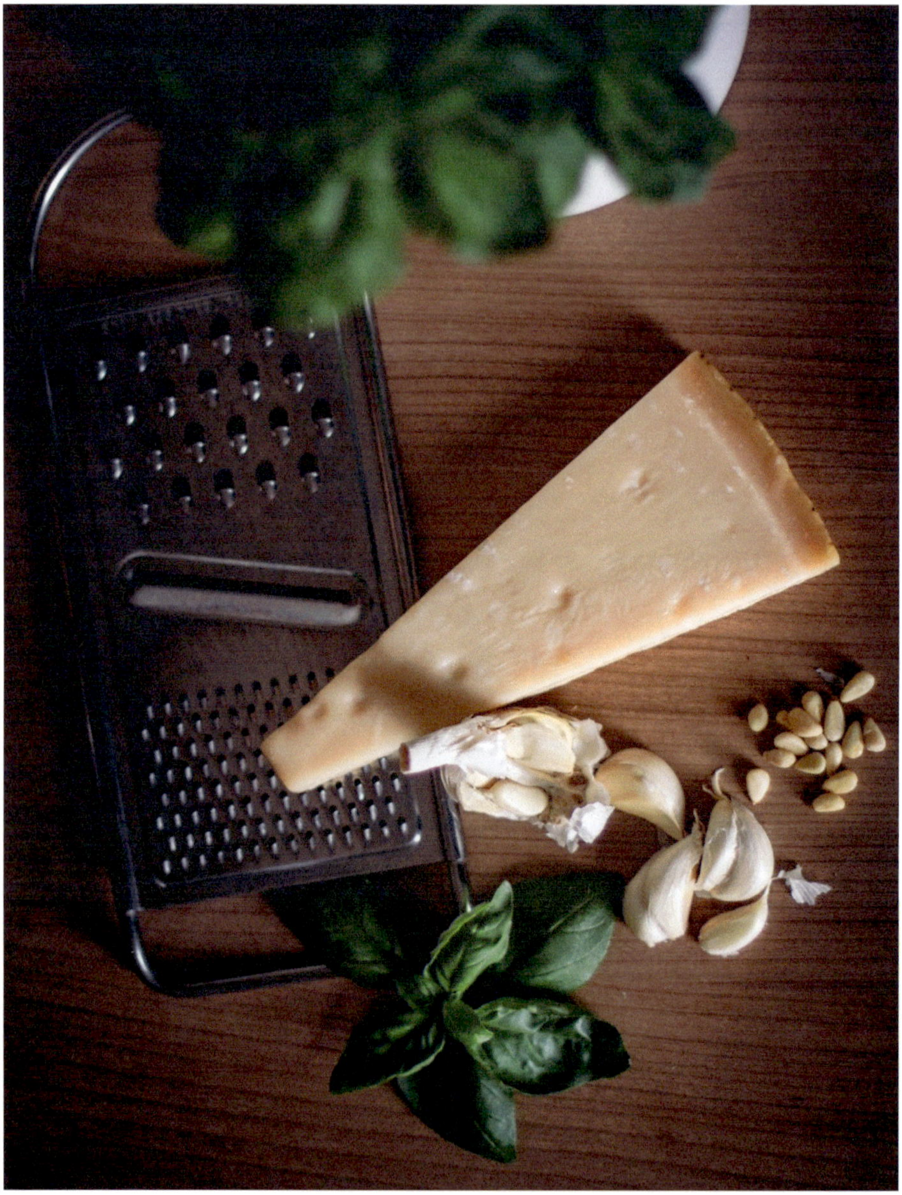

Tuna Patty – high in omega-3

1 can drained Tuna
1 egg white
½ tsp pepper
⅓ cup of low-fat cheddar cheese
½ small onion, finely chopped
1 tsp garlic powder or ¼ tsp minced garlic

1. In a bowl mix all ingredients together until they stick
2. Split in half and form two patties
3. Fry in saucepan until both sides are golden brown

Yield 2 servings, 98 calories; 1.9g fat, 2.1g carbohydrates, 18.3g of protein, 392.5mg sodium

Chili Lime Shrimp - paleo

12 large shrimp, peeled and deveined
1 tbsp olive oil
½ tsp paprika
black pepper to taste
2 tbsp honey
juice 2 limes, save some zest
¼ tsp chili powder
4 skewers

1. Combine oil, zest and lime juice, honey paprika, chili powder and pepper in a bowl
2. Add shrimp to the mixture, coat well
3. Refrigerate and marinate the shrimp for 30minutes, 20 is fine if you are in a rush
4. Cook on a grill for 2-3 minutes per side or in oven at 425°F for 3 minutes per side

Cut the Mustard Loin with Roasted Beets – high protein

2 lbs pork tenderloin
2 tbsp fresh thyme, chopped
¼ cup whole grain Dijon mustard
2 tsp garlic, mined
sea salt and black pepper (season to taste)

1. Preheat oven to 375°F
2. Line a baking sheet with aluminum foil
3. Season pork tenderloin with salt and pepper, place on baking sheet
4. Mix garlic, mustard and thyme together in a small bowl
5. Coat the tenderloin with the mustard mixture, don't forget the sides

6. Roast for 30minutes or until cooked thoroughly
7. Let sit for 10 minutes when done, then serve

Creamy Lime Salmon with Roasted Carrots – high protein

Creamy Lime Dressing

¼ cup honey
¼ cup lime juice, fresh
1 tbsp garlic, minced
1 cup nonfat plain yogurt
1 tbsp ginger, minced
1 tbsp mint, minced
4 4-oz salmon steaks or filets; pacific or Alaskan

1. Combine honey, yogurt, lime juice, ginger, garlic and mint to a glass bowl and wish until creamy. Set half of the dressing aside to serve with cooked salmon
2. Add the salmon to the remaining dressing, cover and refrigerate for 1-2 hours
3. Preheat the oven to 375°F, cook the salmon for 15-20 minutes (20 minutes per inch of thickness; 10 minutes per side)
4. Warm the set aside dressing in a small pan on low for 5-7 minutes towards the 5-10 minutes of salmon cooking
5. Serve warm dressing on the side or drizzled over the roasted carrots

Yield 4, serving size 1 filet, calories 309; 13g fat, 38g carbohydrates, 55g sodium

Roasted Carrots

12 carrots
1¼ tsp sea salt
1½ tbsp olive oil
½ tsp freshly ground black pepper

1. Wash and use a vegetable peeler to remove a thin layer of skin
2. If carrots are thick, cut in half lengthwise, then cut sticks again, should have 4 sticks out of 1 carrot. Toss them in a bowl with the olive oil, salt, and pepper
3. Bake at the same time as the salmon 20minutes, or until desired doneness.

Open Rangoon Style with Sesame Spinach

Olive oil cooking spray
8 ounces lump crab meat
2½ teaspoons curry powder
½ tsp cayenne pepper (optional)
⅓ cup scallions, washed and thinly sliced
24 wonton wrappers
1 tsp Worcestershire sauce
1 tsp ground ginger
½ cup reduced-fat cream cheese

1. Preheat oven to 375°F, and spray mini muffin tin with olive oil spray.
2. Push a wonton wrapper into each muffin tin.
3. In a mixing bowl, combine crab, Worcestershire, curry, ginger, and cayenne.
4. Mix with a fork, breaking up large chunks of crab, then add the cream cheese, mashing with a fork until fully incorporated.
5. Using a teaspoon, spoon filling mixture into wontons.
6. Fold ends of wonton wrapper over mixture, and seal with your finger after dipping in water.
7. Bake for 10 minutes, until ends are slightly browned, and serve hot, garnished with scallions.

Sesame Spinach

1 tbsp toasted sesame seeds (see Tip)
2 tsp reduced-sodium soy sauce or Bragg's Liquid Aminos
2 tsp toasted sesame oil
1 small clove garlic, minced

1. Place water in a very large pot or Dutch oven and bring to a boil over high heat. Add spinach and cook, stirring frequently, until completely wilted, 2 to 3 minutes.
2. Transfer to a colander and let stand until cool enough to handle. Squeeze out excess water.
3. Coarsely chop the spinach. Place in a bowl and mix in sesame seeds, soy sauce, sesame oil and garlic. Serve at room temperature.

21 Cravin'Fit DESSERTS

KEY:

DF – diabetic friendly	**GF** – gluten-free
LC – low carb	**HP** – high protein
P – paleo	**VE** – vegan
VG – vegetarian	

Almond's Joy - vegetarian (exchanges listed for gluten-free, vegan)

1⅓ cup almond flour (such as Bob's Red Mill)
2 ounces dark chocolate, roughly chopped
1 cup shredded coconut, toasted
2 tbsp flaxseed meal
heaping ½ cup pitted dates
⅓ cup maple syrup
¾ cup old-fashioned oats
2 tbsp cocoa powder
1 cup almond butter
2 tsp vanilla extract

1. Add the oats to the bowl of a food processor. Pulse 4-5 times to break up the oats.
2. Add the flaxseed meal, almond flour, shredded coconut, cocoa powder, dark chocolate, and dates to the food processor. Pulse until mixture looks like wet sand. Add the remaining ingredients to the food processor and pulse until mixture begins to form a dough-like ball.
3. Roll the mixture into 1-inch balls, pressing the dough together in the palm of your hand as you roll.
4. Store in an airtight container in the refrigerator for up to two weeks.

Yield 18-20 balls

Cravin'Fit Swaps:

- Gluten-free version use certified gluten-free old-fashioned oats in place of regular oats.
- Vegan, use vegan-friendly cocoa powder and chocolate.

Apple Pecan Crumbs – gluten-free, paleo

6-8 large tart apples, cored, peeled and chopped
½ cup 100% pure maple syrup, will divide for recipe
1 tbsp ground cinnamon
½ tsp ground ginger
4 tbsp coconut oil
Pinch of sea salt, or pink Himalayan salt
½ tsp ground nutmeg
Pinch of cloves
1½ cups finely chopped pecans

1. Preheat oven to 400°F
2. In a large bowl mix apples, ¼ cup maple syrup, cinnamon, nutmeg, ginger, cloves and salt
3. Place mixture in a 9x13 inch baking pan
4. Mix pecans and coconut oil together, until they are crumby and well mixed

5. Stir in the remaining ¼ cup of maple syrup to the crumb mixture
6. Sprinkle the crumbs all over the apple mixture and baked for 30 minutes or until tender
7. Eat it hot and add a dollop of plain non-fat Greek yogurt; it will act as your whipped cream replacement

Blueloupe - diabetic friendly, gluten-free, vegetarian

½ medium cantaloupe, seeded, rind discarded, cut into 4 wedges
½ cup fresh blueberries
1 tbsp fresh mint, chopped
½ tsp grated lime zest
1 tbsp lime juice, freshly squeezed

- Place 2 wedges on 2 plates or meal prep containers, spoon half the berries on each serving. Sprinkle with lime zest, finish by pouring the lime juice over all

Yield 2 servings

Avo-Choco Mousse – gluten-free, paleo,

Recipe requires ripe to very ripe fruit. If you like you can use all organic ingredients and enjoy an organic paleo treat

2 avocados, peeled and pitted
1 large banana
1 cup cocoa powder
½ cup honey
½ cup toasted chopped hazelnuts

1. Place first 4 ingredients in a food processor and pulse until really thick and smooth
2. Spoon into dessert cups, bowls or stemmed glasses
3. Top dessert with hazelnuts and chill in the refrigerator 30mins to an hour

Did Ginger Bark? - vegetarian

¾ cup hazelnuts (about 4 oz)
⅓cup dried cherries, coarsely chopped
2 tbsp finely chopped crystallized ginger
6 oz bittersweet dark chocolate, chopped

1. Preheat oven to 350°F.
2. Place hazelnuts on a baking sheet. Bake at 350°F for 20 minutes, stirring once halfway through cooking. Place nuts on a towel. rub off skins. Coarsely chop nuts. Combine nuts, cherries, and ginger in a medium bowl.
3. Place chocolate in a microwave-safe measuring cup. Microwave at HIGH 1 minute or until chocolate melts, stirring every 15 seconds. Add to nut mixture, stirring just until combined. Spread mixture evenly on a cool or room temperature foil lined pan; freeze 1 hour. Break into pieces; serve immediately.

Coco Bread Pudding - gluten-free, vegetarian

**if you do not require gluten-free, use regular day-old whole grain or wheat bread*

4 cups cubed gluten-free bread, day old and toasted
2 ½ cups fat-free evaporated milk
2 large eggs
⅓ cup unsweetened cocoa powder
⅓ cup light brown sugar
1 tsp vanilla extract

1. Grease a 4-qt slow cooker with non-stick cooking spray. Add the bread cubes
2. In a medium bowl, whish the milk, eggs, sugar, cocoa, and extract until the sugar and cocoa are dissolved. Pour over the bread cubes
3. Cover and cook on low for 5 hours or until the pudding no longer looks wet

Yield 10 servings

Fruit on the Barbie with Yogi Dipping Sauce

¼ honeydew melon, chopped or use a melon baller
¼ cantaloupe, chopped or use a melon baller
1 16oz container of strawberries, sliced
1 apple cut into squares
juice of ½ lemon
1 kiwi, sliced
4-8 skewers

1. Thread fruit on skewers, get creative and alternate fruit
2. Squeeze or sprinkle lemon juice on fruit to preserve freshness

Yield 4-6 kebabs

Yogi Dipping Sauce

2 cups non-fat vanilla Greek yogurt
¼ tsp lemon juice
½ cup honey
½ tsp cinnamon

- Mix all ingredients together in a small bowl

Yield 2 cups (cut recipe in half to make less)

Funky Monkey Chips - vegan

4 medium ripe bananas (or 3 large)
3 tbsp orange juice (or juice from 1 large lemon)
Cinnamon

1. Preheat oven to 200°F (warm setting). Line a baking sheet with parchment paper
2. Peel the bananas and cut into ¼ inch slices. Dip each slice into the orange juice and place on the pan. Sprinkle with cinnamon.
3. Bake for 3 to 4 hours, or until your chips are dry and slightly brown, making sure to flip your chips halfway through.
4. Remove from the oven, and once cool, chips can be stored in an airtight container.

Yield 2, 148 calories

Mango Ice Cream – gluten-free, vegetarian , vegan

1 cup frozen mango chunks
2 frozen bananas, peels removed prior to freezing
Dark chocolate (optional, for garnish), gluten-free

1. Slice the bananas and place them in a blender or food processor with the frozen mango.
2. Blend until smooth and enjoy immediately as is or topped with dark chocolate shavings.

Yield 2 servings, 150 calories

Orange Broil – gluten-free, vegetarian

2 medium oranges
2 tbsp slivered/sliced almonds or pecans
½ tsp ground cinnamon
2 packets of stevia

1. Preheat the broiler line a small baking tray or pan
2. Peel oranges over bowl to save the juice
3. Over a bowl, cut the oranges in round slices about ½ inch thick
4. Arrange slices in a single layer on the pan or dish. Sprinkle with cinnamon and almonds and broil for 3 minutes
5. Add the stevia packets to the reserved juice, stir to combine and dissolve. Pour over the broiled oranges and serve
6. Feel free to add a dollop of fat-free Greek yogurt

Gorgonzola Figs – low carb, vegetarian

4 medium fresh figs
¼ cup Gorgonzola, crumbled
½ cup walnuts, walnuts

1. Slice the figs in half, spread each half with a tablespoon of Gorgonzola, and sprinkle with ½ tbsp chopped walnuts
2. Feel free to broil your figs for a few minutes first.

Yield 4 servings of 2 halves, 12g carbohydrates, 2g fiber, 9g protein

Pineapple Mint Smoothie – gluten-free, paleo

1 cup pineapple chunks
1 tbsp raw natural honey
8-9 ice cubes
1 ½ cup green tea, room temp
8 mint leaves
Few drops of vanilla extract

- Blend all ingredients until smooth, or desired consistency

PB Banana Folds - vegetarian

1 package of egg roll wraps, (Try Nasoya mini)
¼ cup peanut butter or almond/cashew butter
Dash of cinnamon
2 bananas sliced
1 tsp coconut oil melted

1. Place one slice of banana and 1 tsp of peanut butter in each wrap with a dash of cinnamon
2. Using water on your fingers, wrap in desired shape, triangles work well, and seal
3. Lightly brush tops with coconut oil
4. Place on parchment paper lined baking sheet and bake at 400°F for 10-15 minutes or until golden brown
5. Enjoy with dark chocolate dipping sauce (melt dark chocolate mixed with 1 tsp of coconut oil)

Raspberry Power bowl - gluten-free, vegetarian

¼ cup cooked quinoa (56 calories)
⅓ cup nonfat Greek yogurt (45 calories)
2 tbsp raw almonds (78 calories)
1 tbsp raspberry preserves (40 calories)

- Assemble first 3 ingredients and top with raspberry preserve

Yield 1 serving, 219 calories

Poached Pears - gluten-free, low carb, vegetarian

4 Bosc pears, peeled
2 tbsp vanilla extract
1 vanilla bean, split
2 cups of water

1. Stand pears upright in a 4qt slow cooker, then add remaining ingredients
2. Cook on low for 2 hours or until tender

3. *Tip:* to get pears to stand up right, cut the bottoms straight across to level

Yield 4

Pineapple Dreams - vegan

2 cups frozen pineapple
½ frozen banana
2 tbsp unsweetened almond milk

1. Place all three ingredients in the blender or food processor and turn it on. Every minute or so, stop and scrape down the sides.
2. After several minutes, you should have an evenly creamy consistency.
3. Spoon it into your dish, or get fancy with a piping bag and a star nozzle, and swirl it all around.
4. Enjoy on its own, or top with sliced strawberries, a bit of unsweetened shredded coconut, or a few chocolate chips.

Strawberry Banana Ice Cream - gluten-free, paleo, vegetarian

3 frozen bananas, (frozen when really ripe)
½ cup coconut cream, or full-fat coconut milk
1 cup strawberries, frozen
1 tsp vanilla extract

- Process in a food processor for 1-2 minutes until its smooth like soft serve ice cream

Yield 4 servings, 135 calories

Tangy Quats - gluten-free, vegetarian

½ cup cooked quinoa (111 calories)
1 tbsp honey (64 calories)
2 oz kumquats (40 calories) or figs
2 oz pomegranate seeds (24 calories)

- Top quinoa with kumquats, pomegranate seeds and drizzle with honey

Yield 1 serving, 239 calories

Mrs. Maple's Nut – gluten-free, paleo, vegan

2 tbsp pure maple syrup; *if you have vegan concerns look for a Kosher brand*
6 oz raw walnuts
½ tsp kosher salt
1 tbsp melted coconut oil
¼ tsp cayenne pepper

1. Preheat the oven to 350°F
2. Add walnuts, syrup, melted oil, salt and cayenne to a bowl and stir to combine and coat the nuts well. Spread them in a single layer on a baking sheet lined with parchment paper
3. Bake the nuts on the middle rack for 15 minutes, stir often for even cooking. Check at the 10 minutes mark to prevent burning
4. Take the walnuts out of the oven, and give them one final toss. They will be sticky, the coating will harden as the nuts cool.

Yield ¾ cup

Sour Berry Parfait – low sugar

1 cup of berries (*select or mix your selection to equal one cup*) strawberry, blueberry, raspberry or blackberry
½ cup lemon yogurt
¼ cup no/low-fat whipped topping

1. In a small bowl fold in the whipped topping with the yogurt
2. Put ½ cup berries in the bottom of 2 dessert cups (¼ cup per dessert cup)
3. Split the yogurt mixture between the cups, top with the remaining berries

Yield 2 servings, 83 calories; 17g carbohydrates, 2g fiber, 3g protein

Hot Chocolate - gluten-free, vegetarian

1 cup vanilla almond milk or soymilk
4 tbsp cocoa powder
1 tsp honey

1. Mix milk and honey in your favorite mug, microwave for 1 minute
2. Stir in the cocoa powder to mix the honey and powder
3. Enjoy immediately

BIBLIOGRAPHY

Allen, James. *As A Man Thinketh*. N.p.: Tribecca, 1903. 27-53. Print.

Borushek, Allan. *Calorie, Fat & Carbohydrate Counter: Plus 200 Fast-food Chains & Restaurants*. Costa Mesa, CA: Family Health Publications, 2007. Print.

Brynie, Faith Hickman. *101 Questions About Food and Digestion*. Brookfield: Twenty-First Century, 2002. Print.

Burke, Cindy. *To Buy or Not to Buy Organic: What You Need to Know to Choose the Healthiest, Safest, Most Earth-friendly Food*. New York, NY: Marlowe, 2007. 157-78. Print.

Carboni, Camilla, and Melissa Van Dover. *Paleo Cleanse: 30 Days of Ancestral Eating to Detox, Drop Pounds, Supercharge Your Health and Transition into a Primal Lifestyle*. Berkely: Ulysses, 2014. Print.

Coffey, Linda, and Ann H. Baier. *USDA Guide for Organic Livestock Producers*. N.p.: National Center for Appropriate Technology (NCAT) Agriculture Specialists, Nov. 2012. PDF. https://www.ams.usda.gov/sites/default/files/media/Guide for Organic Livestock Producers_0.pdf

Dunn-Lewis, Courtenay, M.A., and William Kraemer, Ph.D., FACSM. "*The Basics of Starting and Progressing a Strength-Training Program*." ACSM. American College of Sports Medicine, 13 Jan. 2012. Web. 5 Mar. 2016. <http://www.acsm.org/public-information/articles/2012/01/13/the-basics-of-starting-and-progressing-a-strength-training-program>.

"Food Irradiation: What You Need to Know." *Food Irradiation: What You Need to Know*. US Dept of Health and Human Services, 3 Sept. 2015. Web. 2 Feb. 2016. <http://www.fda.gov/Food/ResourcesForYou/Consumers/ucm261680.htm>.

Gilmore, Megan, and Nicole Franzen. *Everyday Detox: 100 Easy Recipes to Remove Toxins, Promote Gut Health, and Lose Weight Naturally*. 1st ed. N.p.:

Ten Speed, 2015. Print.

"How to Understand and Use the Nutrition Facts Label." *U.S. Food and Drug Administration*. U.S. Department of Health and Human Services, 30 Nov. 2015. Web. 12 Feb. 2016. <http://www.fda.gov/Food/IngredientsPackagingLabeling/LabelingNutrition/ucm274593.htm>.

Lawless, Annie. *The Suja Juice Solution: 7 Days to Lose Fat, Beat Cravings, and Boost Your Energy*. 1st ed. New York: Grand Central Life & Style, 2015. Print.

Nania, Rachel. "What You Need to Know about Farm-raised vs. Wild-caught Fish." *WTOP*. WTOP, 2 June 2015. Web. 30 Jan. 2016. <http://wtop.com/food/2015/06/what-you-need-to-know-about-farm-raised-vs-wild-caught-fish/>.

Newman, Joni-Marie, and Gerrie Lynn Adams. *Going Vegan: The Complete Guide to Making a Healthy Transition to a Plant-based Lifestyle*. Beverly: Fair Winds, 2014. Print.

Oz, Daphne. *The Dorm Room Diet: The 8-step Program for Creating a Healthy Lifestyle Plan That Really Works*. New York: Newmarket, 2006. Print.

Olender, Katherine. "8 Trick-Free Ways To Know What You're Eating." *Food Insight*. International Food Information Council Foundation, 24 July 2014. Web. 12 Feb. 2016. <http://www.foodinsight.org/blogs/8-trick-free-ways-know-what-youre-eating>.

Pedersen, Stephanie. *The 7-day Superfood Cleanse*. New York: Sterling, 2015. Print.

Pratt, Steven, and Kathy Matthews. *Superfoods Healthstyle: Achieve Total Health and Rejuvenation for the Rest of Your Life*. First ed. New York: Morrow, 2006. Print.

Terry, Bryant. *Afro-vegan: Farm-fresh African, Caribbean & Southern Flavors Remixed*. Berkeley: Ten Speed, n.d. 126, 181. Print.

Tracy, Tennille. "House Votes to Remove Country-of-Origin Labels on Meat Sold in U.S." *The Wall Street Journal*. The Wall Street Journal, 10 June 2015. Web. 5 Jan. 2016. <http://www.wsj.com/articles/house-votes-to-remove-country-of-origin-labels-on-meat-sold-in-u-s-1433990294>.

Westen, Robin. *The Metabolism-boost Cleanse: A 3-day Detox to Reset Your System for Maximum Health, Energy and Fat Burning*. N.p.: n.p., n.d. Print.

Woodruff, Sandra L. *Secrets of Good-carb/low-carb Living*. New York: Avery, 2004. Print.

Zimelman, Elana, RD, LD, CDE. "Clearing up Food Label Confusion." *Living Well Magazine, Dallas County* Jan/Feb. 2016: 20-21. Print.

ABOUT THE AUTHOR

Velma D. Canaday, is a Certified Nutritionist awarded by The American Fitness Professional Association. Velma is a Wellness Advisor at Pure Plates in Dallas, Texas where she currently resides. She is also the owner of a legging and yoga pant apparel business; Tights Presented by Velma Canaday.

For more information visit www.VelmaCanaday.com and to visit her legging apparel business visit shop.VelmaCanaday.com.

Supplemental information for the book can be found at www.VelmaCanaday.com/21CravinFit.html.